AN ILLUSTRATED COLOUR

DERMATOLOGY

DAVID J. GAWKRODGER MD FRCP FRCPE

Consultant Dermatologist and Honorary Clinical Lecturer,
University of Sheffield,
Royal Hallamshire Hospital,
Sheffield, UK

SECOND EDITION

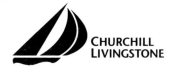

CHURCHILL LIVINGSTONE

NEW YORK EDINBURGH LONDON MADRID MELBOURNE SAN FRANCISCO TOKYO 1997

CHURCHILL LIVINGSTONE
Medical Division of Longman Group UK Limited

Distributed in the United States of America by
Churchill Livingstone Inc., 650 Avenue of the Americas, New York,
N.Y. 10011 and by associated companies, branches and representatives throughout the world.

© Pearson Professional 1997 © Longman Group UK Limited 1992,
assigned to Pearson Professional 1995

The right of Dr David Gawkrodger to be identified as author of this
work has been asserted by him in accordance with the Copyright,
Designs and Patents Act 1988.

First edition published 1992
Second edition published 1997

ISBN 0-443-053286

British Library Cataloguing in Publication Data
A catalogue record for this book is available from the British Library.

Library of Congress Cataloging in Publication Data
A catalog record for this book is available from the Library of Congress.

Medical knowledge is constantly changing. As new information
becomes available, changes in treatment, procedures, equipment and
the use of drugs become necessary. The author and the publishers
have, as far as it is possible, taken care to ensure that the information
given in this text is accurate and up to date. However, readers are
strongly advised to confirm that the information, especially with
regard to drug usage, complies with current legislation and standards
of practice.

For Churchill Livingstone

Publisher: Timothy Horne
Project manager: Ninette Premdas
Design: Sarah Cape
Project controller: Kay Hunston

Produced by Longman Asia Ltd, Hong Kong
SWT/01

The
publisher's
policy is to use
**paper manufactured
from sustainable forests**

PREFACE TO THE SECOND EDITION

Dermatology texts are either too long, too short, or too simplistic in the visually descriptive sense. To find a compromise between the reader's desire for brevity and the need to provide sufficient detail of mechanisms has not been easy, but I hope that the balance in this book is about right.

In making changes and additions for the second edition, I have taken account of recent developments, e.g. in molecular genetics and HIV disease, and emphasized additional areas of importance, e.g. the skin in old age and occupational dermatoses. The new edition has allowed me to improve illustrations, correct long-established but incorrect truisms, and reflect the therapeutic dogmas of today.

Sheffield
1997

David J. Gawkrodger

PREFACE TO THE FIRST EDITION

Recent advances in publishing technology and book presentation demand that a modern text be attractively and concisely presented, in colour and at an affordable price. This is essential for success in a very competitive market. In writing this book, I have attempted to present an introductory dermatology text for the 1990s, using a format of individually designed double-page spreads, generously illustrated with colour photographs, line drawings, tables, bulleted items and 'key point' summaries. This unique approach, which deals with each topic as an educational unit, allows the reader better accessibility to the facts and greater ease in revision than is possible with a conventional textbook.

The book is aimed at medical students but contains sufficient detail to be of use to family practitioners, physicians in internal medicine, registrars or residents in dermatoloty, and dermatological nurses. The contents are divided into three sections. The first presents a scientific basis for the understanding of and clinical approach to skin disease. The second details the major dermatological conditions, and the third outlines special topics, such as photoageing and dermatological surgery, that are of current importance or that are poorly dealt with in other textbooks.

Sheffield
1992

David J. Gawkrodger

ACKNOWLEDGEMENTS

In the production of the second edition of this book it is a pleasure to acknowledge the contribution of the publishing staff at Churchill Livingstone, particularly Ninette Premdas, project manager and Sarah Cape, senior designer. I am very grateful to the following colleagues who gave helpful advice about improving the content of the book: Dr M.M. Black, Professor J.L. Burton, Professor R.D.R. Camp, Dr G.B. Colver, Dr N.H. Cox, Dr R.P.R. Dawber, Professor R.A.J. Eady, Dr J.S.C. English, Dr A.Y. Finlay, Professor C.E.M. Griffiths, Professor J.A.A. Hunter, Dr G.R. Kinghorn, Dr M. Makris, Dr R. Murphy, Professor T.J. Ryan, Dr J.A. Savin, Professor S. Shuster, Dr F.J. Storrs and Dr M.D. Talbot. I also thank my secretary Mrs G.K. Sykes for her hard work on many tasks.

Several of the new illustrations have been kindly and generously provided by colleagues and I thank Dr E.C. Benton of Edinburgh, Dr J.E. Bothwell of Barnsley, Dr J.S.C. Englishof Nottingham, Dr F.M. Lewis of Worcester, Dr S.M. Morley of Dundee, and Professor S.S. Bleehen, Mr D. Dobbs, Dr C.I. Harrington, Dr A.J.G. McDonagh, Dr A.G. Messenger, Mr G. Ravichandran, Dr M. Shah and Dr C. Yeoman of Sheffield. Figure 2 (p. 26) is reproduced by permission of the British Medical Association (originally used in ABC of Dermatology by P.K. Buxton, 1988) and figure 2 (p. 16) is reproduced by permission of Blackwell Science (originally used in Clinical Dermatology by J.A.A. Hunter, J.A. Savin and M.V. Dahl, 1989). Figure 4 (p. 101) is reproduced courtesy of the editor of the British Journal of Dermatology and Dr E.F. Bernstein of Jefferson Medical College, Philadelphia, USA. Figures 2 and 4 (p. 114) are reproduced courtesy of Blackwell Science (having originally appeared in the Textbook of Dermatology, fifth edition, edited by R.H. Champion, J.L. Burton, F.J.G. Ebling, 1992). I am grateful to the following for advice or for the provision of illustrations: Professor R. Barnetston, Dr G.W. Beveridge, Dr P.K. Buxton, the late Professor F.J.G. Ebling, Dr M.E. Kesseler, Dr C. McGibbon, Dr A. McMillan, Mrs E. McVittie, Dr C.O'Doherty, Miss M.J. Spencer and Dr A.E. Walker. I also thank those patients who gave permission for their faces to be shown without eyebars.

Sheffield 1997
David J. Gawkrodger

CONTENTS

BASIC
PRINCIPLES

MICROANATOMY OF THE SKIN

INTRODUCTION

The skin is one of the largest organs in the body, having a surface area of $1.8\,m^2$ and making up about 16% of body weight. It has many functions, the most important of which is as a barrier to protect the body from noxious external factors and to keep the internal systems intact.

Skin is composed of three layers: the epidermis, the dermis and the subcutis (Fig. 1).

EPIDERMIS

The epidermis is defined as a stratified squamous epithelium which is about 0.1 mm thick, although the thickness is greater (0.8–1.4 mm) on the palm and sole. Its prime function is to act as a protective barrier. The main cell of the epidermis is the *keratinocyte*, which produces the protein keratin. The four layers of the epidermis (Fig. 2) represent the stages of maturation of keratin by keratinocytes (p. 6).

Basal cell layer (stratum basale)

The basal cell layer of the epidermis is comprised mostly of keratinocytes which are either dividing or non-dividing. The cells contain keratin tonofibrils (p. 6) and are secured to the basement membrane (Fig. 2) by hemidesmosomes. *Melanocytes* make up 5–10% of the basal cell population. These cells synthesize melanin (p. 8) and transfer it via dendritic processes to neighbouring keratinocytes. Melanocytes are most numerous on the face and other exposed sites and are of neural crest origin. *Merkel cells* are also found, albeit infrequently, in the basal cell layer. These cells are closely associated with terminal filaments of cutaneous nerves and seem to have a role in sensation. Their cytoplasm contains neuropeptide granules, as well as neurofilaments and keratin.

Prickle cell layer (stratum spinosum)

Daughter basal cells migrate upwards to form this layer of polyhedral cells which are interconnected by desmosomes (the 'prickles' seen at light microscope level). Keratin tonofibrils form a supportive mesh in the cytoplasm of these cells. *Langerhans cells* are found mostly in this layer; these dendritic, immunologically active cells are fully described on page 10.

Granular cell layer (stratum granulosum)

Cells become flattened and lose their nuclei in the granular cell layer. Keratohyalin granules are seen in the cytoplasm together with membrane-coating granules (which expel their lipid contents into the intercellular spaces).

Fig. 1 **Structure of the skin.** The diagram shows a comparison between thick, hairless skin (plantar and palmar) and thinner, hirsute skin.

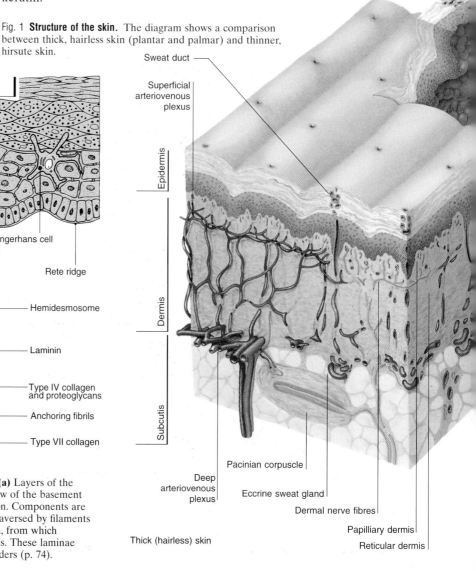

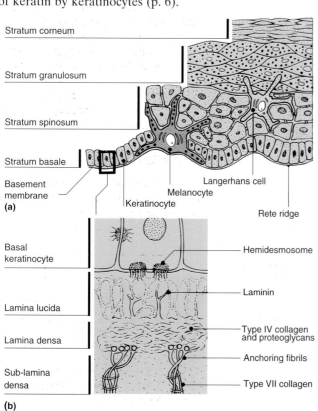

Fig. 2 **Cross-sectional anatomy of the epidermis. (a)** Layers of the epidermis and other structures. **(b)** Detailed view of the basement membrane zone at the dermo-epidermal junction. Components are arranged in three layers. The lamina lucida is traversed by filaments connecting the basal cells with the lamina densa, from which anchoring fibrils extend into the papillary dermis. These laminae are the sites of cleavage in certain bullous disorders (p. 74).

EMBRYOLOGY OF THE SKIN

The epidermis (ectoderm) begins to develop at four weeks of life, and by seven weeks, flat cells overlying the basal layer form the periderm (which is eventually cast off). Nails start to take shape at 10 weeks. The dermis (mesoderm) develops at 11 weeks, and by 12 weeks, indented basal buds of the epidermis form the hair bulbs, with dermal papillae supplying vessels and nerves. Fingerprint ridges are determined by 17 weeks gestation.

Horny layer (stratum corneum)

The end result of keratinocyte maturation can be found in the horny layer which is comprised of sheets of overlapping polyhedral cornified cells with no nuclei (corneocytes). The layer is several cells thick on the palms and soles, but less thick elsewhere. The corneocyte cell envelope is broadened, and the cytoplasm is replaced by keratin tonofibrils in a matrix formed from the keratohyalin granules. Cells are stuck together by a lipid glue which is partly derived from membrane-coating granules.

DERMIS

The dermis is defined as a tough supportive connective tissue matrix, containing specialized structures, found immediately below and intimately connected with the epidermis. It varies in thickness, being thin (0.6 mm) on the eyelids and thicker (3 mm or more) on the back, palms and soles. The *papillary dermis* — the thin upper layer of the dermis — lies below and interdigitates with the epidermal rete ridges. It is composed of loosely interwoven collagen. Coarser and horizontally running bundles of collagen are found in the deeper and thicker *reticular dermis*.

Collagen fibres make up 70% of the dermis and impart a toughness and strength to the structure. *Elastin* fibres are loosely arranged in all directions in the dermis and provide elasticity to the skin. They are numerous near hair follicles and sweat glands, and less so in the papillary dermis. The *ground substance* of the dermis is a semi-solid matrix of glycosaminoglycans (GAG) which allows dermal structures some movement (p. 9).

The dermis contains fibroblasts (which synthesize collagen, elastin, other connective tissue and GAG), dermal dendrocytes (dendritic cells with a probable immune function), mast cells, macrophages and lymphocytes.

SUBCUTANEOUS LAYER

The subcutis consists of loose connective tissue and fat (up to 3 cm thick on the abdomen).

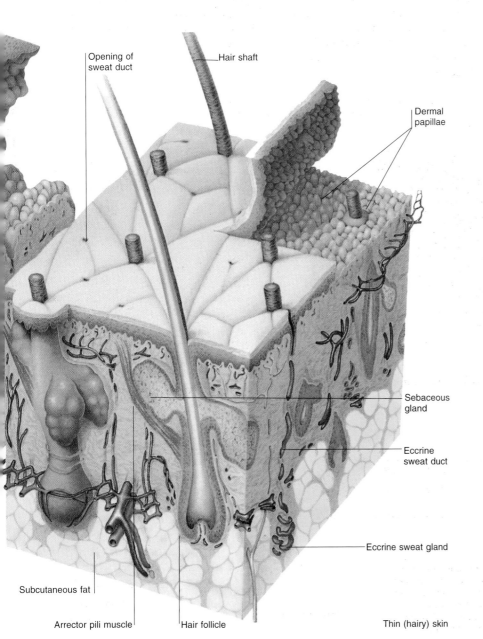

Opening of sweat duct

Hair shaft

Dermal papillae

Sebaceous gland

Eccrine sweat duct

Eccrine sweat gland

Subcutaneous fat

Arrector pili muscle

Hair follicle

Thin (hairy) skin

Microanatomy

- The skin comprises 16% of body weight; surface area 1.8 m².
- Structure and thickness vary with site.
- The epidermis is the outer covering, mainly composed of keratinocytes arranged in four layers.
- The dermis is supportive connective tissue, mainly collagen, elastin and glycosaminoglycans.

DERIVATIVES OF THE SKIN

HAIR

Hairs are found over the entire surface of the skin, with the exception of the glabrous skin of the palms, soles, glans penis and vulval introitus. The density of follicles is greatest on the face. Embryologically, the hair follicle has an input from the epidermis, which is responsible for the matrix cells and the hair shaft, and the dermis, which contributes the papilla, with its blood vessels, and nerves.

There are three types of hair:

- *Lanugo* hairs are fine and long, and are formed in the fetus at 20 weeks gestation. They are normally shed before birth, but may be seen in premature babies.
- *Vellus* hairs are the short, fine, light coloured hairs that cover most body surfaces.
- *Terminal* hairs are longer, thicker and darker and are found on the scalp, eyebrows, eyelashes, and also on the pubic, axillar and beard areas. They originate as vellus hair; differentiation is stimulated at puberty by androgens.

STRUCTURE

The hair shaft consists of an *outer cuticle* which encloses a cortex of packed keratinocytes with (in terminal hairs) an *inner medulla* (Fig. 1). The germinative cells are in the hair bulb; associated with these cells are melanocytes which synthesize pigment. The *arrector pili* muscle is vestigial in man; it contracts with cold, fear and emotion to erect the hair, producing 'goose pimples'.

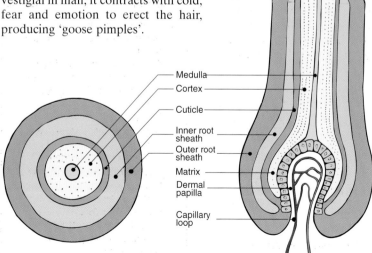

Fig. 1 **Structure of the hair follicle.**

NAILS

The nail is a phylogenetic remnant of the mammalian claw and consists of a plate of hardened and densely packed keratin. It protects the finger tip and facilitates grasping and tactile sensitivity in the finger pulp.

STRUCTURE

The *nail matrix* contains dividing cells which mature, keratinize and move forward to form the *nail plate* (Fig. 2). The nail plate has a thickness of 0.3–0.5 mm and grows at a rate of 0.1 mm/24h for the fingernail. Toenails grow more slowly. The *nail bed*, which produces small amounts of keratin, is adherent to the nail plate. The adjacent dermal capillaries produce the pink colour of the nail; the white lunula is the visible distal part of the matrix. The *hyponychium* is the thickened epidermis which underlies the free margin of the nail.

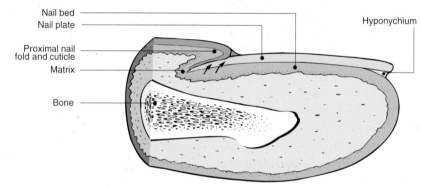

Fig. 2 **Structure of the fingernail.**

SEBACEOUS GLANDS

Sebaceous glands are found associated with hair follicles (Fig. 3), especially those of the scalp, face, chest and back, and are not found on non-hairy skin. They are formed from epidermis-derived cells and produce an oily sebum, the function of which is uncertain.

The glands are small in the child but become large and active at puberty, being sensitive to androgens. Sebum is produced by holocrine secretion in which the cells disintegrate to release their lipid cytoplasm.

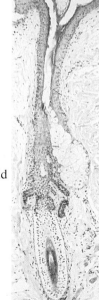

Fig. 3 **Sebaceous gland in association with a hair follicle.** The gland becomes active at puberty.

SWEAT GLANDS

Sweat glands (Fig. 4) are tube-like and coiled glands, located within the dermis, which produce a watery secretion. There are two separate types: eccrine and apocrine.

ECCRINE

Eccrine sweat glands develop from down budding of the epidermis. The secretory portion is a coiled structure in the deep reticular dermis; the excretory duct spirals upwards to open onto the skin surface. An estimated 2.5 million sweat ducts are present on the skin surface. They are universally distributed but are most profuse on the palms, soles, axillae and forehead where the glands are under both psychological and thermal control (those elsewhere being under thermal control only). Eccrine sweat glands are innervated by sympathetic (cholinergic) nerve fibres.

APOCRINE

Also derived from the epidermis, apocrine sweat glands open into hair follicles and are larger than eccrine glands. They are most numerous around the axillae, perineum and areolae. Their sweat is generated by 'decapitation' secretion of the gland's cells and is odourless when produced; an odour develops after skin bacteria have acted upon it. Sweating is controlled by sympathetic (adrenergic) innervation. The apocrine glands represent a phylogenetic remnant of the mammalian sexual scent gland.

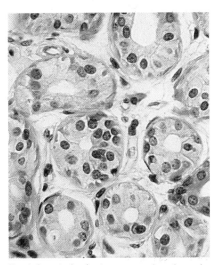

Fig. 4 **Sweat gland.** A cross-section through the coiled secretory portion of an eccrine sweat gland, situated deep in the dermis.

OTHER STRUCTURES IN SKIN

NERVE SUPPLY

The skin is richly innervated (Fig. 5), with the highest density of nerves being found in areas such as the hands, face and genitalia. All nerves supplying the skin have their cell bodies in the dorsal root ganglia. Both myelinated and non-myelinated fibres are found. The nerves contain neuropeptides e.g. substance P.

Free sensory nerve endings are seen in the dermis and also encroaching into the epidermis where they may abut onto *Merkel cells*. These nerve endings detect pain, itch and temperature. Specialized corpuscular receptors are distributed in the dermis, such as the *Pacinian corpuscle* (detecting pressure and vibration) and the touch-sensitive *Meissner's corpuscles* which are mainly seen in the dermal papillae of the feet and hands.

Autonomic nerves supply the blood vessels, sweat glands and arrector pili muscles. The nerve supply is dermatomal with some overlap.

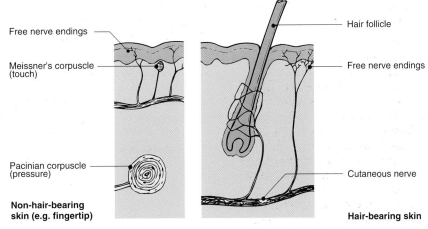

Free nerve endings
Meissner's corpuscle (touch)
Pacinian corpuscle (pressure)
Non-hair-bearing skin (e.g. fingertip)

Hair follicle
Free nerve endings
Cutaneous nerve
Hair-bearing skin

Fig. 5 **Nerve supply to the skin.**

BLOOD AND LYMPHATIC VESSELS

The skin also has a rich and adaptive blood supply. Arteries in the subcutis branch upwards, forming a superficial plexus at the papillary/reticular dermal boundary. Branches extend to the dermal papillae (Fig. 6), each of which has a single loop of capillary vessels, one arterial and one venous. Veins drain from the venous side of this loop to form the mid-dermal and subcutaneous venous networks. In the reticular and papillary dermis there are arteriovenous anastomoses which are well innervated and concerned with thermoregulation (see p. 7).

The lymphatic drainage of the skin is important, and abundant meshes of lymphatics originate in the papillae and assemble into larger vessels which ultimately drain into the regional lymph nodes.

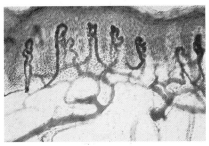

Fig. 6 **Superficial dermal blood vessels.** Capillary loops branch off the superficial vascular plexus and extend into each dermal papilla.

Derivatives

- Sebaceous glands, associated with hair follicles, are androgen-sensitive.
- Vellus hairs cover most body surfaces; terminal hairs occur on scalp, beard, axillar and pubic areas.
- Skin has extensive nerve networks with specialized nerve endings.
- Skin has a rich and adaptive blood supply; lymphatics drain to regional lymph nodes.
- Eccrine sweat glands, with sympathetic innervation, are under thermal/psychological control; apocrine glands are largely vestigial in humans.

PHYSIOLOGY OF THE SKIN

The skin is a metabolically active organ with vital functions (Table 1) including the protection and homeostasis of the body.

Table 1 **Functions of skin**

Presents barrier to physical agents
Protects against mechanical injury
Prevents loss of body fluids
Reduces penetration of UV radiation
Helps regulate body temperature
Acts as a sensory organ
Affords a surface for grip
Plays a role in Vitamin D production
Acts as an outpost for immune surveillance
Cosmetic association

KERATINOCYTE MATURATION

The differentiation of basal cells into dead, but functionally important, corneocytes is a unique feature of the skin. The horny layer is important in preventing all manner of agents from entering the skin, including microorganisms, water and particulate matter. The epidermis also prevents the body's fluids from getting out.

Epidermal cells undergo the following sequence during keratinocyte maturation (Fig. 1).

1. Undifferentiated cells in the **basal layer** and the layer immediately above divide continuously. Half of these cells remain in place and half progress upwards and differentiate.

2. In the **prickle cell layer**, cells change from being columnar to polygonal. Differentiating keratinocytes synthesize keratins which aggregate to form tonofilaments. The *desmosomes* connecting keratinocytes are condensations of tonofilaments. Desmosomes distribute structural stresses throughout the epidermis and maintain a distance of 20 nm between adjacent cells.

3. In the **granular layer**, enzymes induce degradation of nuclei and organelles. Keratohyalin granules mature the keratin and provide an amorphous protein matrix for the tonofilaments. Membrane-coating granules attach to the cell membrane and release an impervious lipid containing cement which contributes to cell adhesion and to the *horny layer* barrier.

4. In the **horny layer**, the dead, flattened corneocytes have developed thickened cell envelopes encasing a matrix of keratin tonofibrils. The strong disulphide bonds of the keratin provide strength to the stratum corneum, but the layer is also flexible and can absorb up to three times its own weight in water. However, if it dries out (i.e. water content falls below 10%), pliability fails.

5. The corneocytes are eventually shed from the skin surface.

RATE OF MATURATION

Kinetic studies show that, on average, the dividing basal cells replicate every 200 to 400 hours, and the resultant differentiating cells take about 14 days to reach the stratum corneum and a further 14 days to be shed. The cell turnover time is considerably shortened in keratinization disorders such as psoriasis.

HAIR GROWTH

In most mammals, hair or fur plays an essential role in survival, especially in the conservation of heat; this is not the case in 'nude' humans. Scalp hair in humans does function as a protection against the cancer-inducing effects of ultraviolet radiation; it also protects against minor injury. However, the main role of hair in human society is as an organ of sexual attraction, and therein lies its importance to the cosmetics industry.

The rate of hair growth differs depending on the site. For example, eyebrow hair grows faster and has a shorter anagen (see below) than scalp hair. On average, there are about 100 000 hairs on the scalp, and the normal rate of growth is 0.4 mm/24 h. Hair growth is cyclical, with three phases, and is randomized for individual hairs, although synchronization does occur during pregnancy. The three phases of hair development (Fig. 2) are anagen, catagen and telogen.

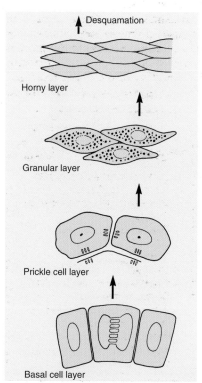

Fig. 1 **Keratinocyte maturation.**

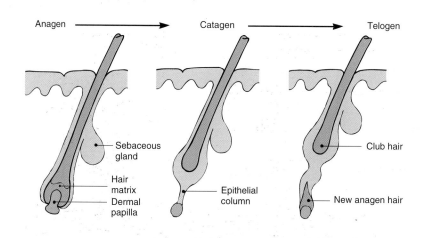

Fig. 2 **The three phases of hair development.**

1. **Anagen** is the growing phase. For scalp hair this lasts from 3–7 years, but for eyebrow hair it lasts only 4 months. At any one time, 80–90% of scalp hairs are in anagen, and about 50–100 scalp follicles switch to catagen per day.

2. **Catagen** is the resting phase and lasts 3–4 weeks. Hair protein synthesis stops and the follicle retreats towards the surface. At any one time 10–20% of scalp hairs are in catagen.

3. **Telogen** is the shedding phase, distinguished by the presence of hairs with a short club root. Each day 50–100 scalp hairs are shed, with less than 1% of hairs being in telogen at any one time.

MELANOCYTE FUNCTION

Melanocytes (located in the basal layer) produce the pigment melanin in elongated, membrane-bound organelles known as melanosomes

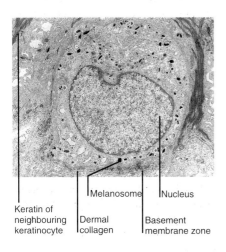

Fig. 3 **Electronmicrograph of a melanocyte.**

(Fig. 3). These are packaged into granules which are moved down dendritic processes and transferred by phagocytosis to adjacent keratinocytes. Melanin granules form a protective cap over the outer part of keratinocyte nuclei in the inner layers of the epidermis. In the stratum corneum, they are uniformly distributed to form a UV-absorbing blanket which reduces the amount of radiation penetrating the skin.

UV radiation — mainly the wavelengths of 290 to 320nm (UVB) — darkens the skin firstly by immediate photo-oxidation of preformed melanin, and secondly over a period of days by stimulating melanocytes to produce more melanin. UV radiation also induces keratinocyte proliferation, resulting in thickening of the epidermis.

Variations in racial pigmentation are due not to differences in melanocyte numbers, but to the number and size of melanosomes produced. Red-haired people have phaeomelanin, not the more usual eumelanin (p. 8), and their melanosomes are spherical rather than oblong.

THERMOREGULATION

The maintenance of a near-constant body core temperature of 37°C is a great advantage to humans, allowing a constancy to many biochemical reactions which would otherwise fluctuate widely with temperature changes. Thermoregulation depends on several factors, including metabolism and exercise, but the skin plays an important part in control through the evaporation of sweat and by direct heat loss from the surface.

BLOOD FLOW

Skin temperature is highly responsive to skin blood flow. Dilation or contraction of the dermal blood vessels results in vast changes in blood flow, which can vary from 1–100ml/min per 100g of skin for the fingers and forearms. Arteriovenous anastomoses under the control of the sympathetic nervous system shunt blood to the superficial venous plexuses (Fig. 4), affecting skin temperature. Local factors, both chemical and physical, can also have an effect.

SWEAT

The production of sweat cools the skin through evaporation. The minimum insensible perspiration per day is 0.5 litre. Maximum daily secretion is 10 litres, with a maximum output of about 2 litres per hour. Men sweat more than women.

Watery isotonic sweat, produced in the sweat gland, is modified in the excretory portion of the duct so that the fluid delivered to the skin surface has:

- a pH of between 4 and 6.8
- a low concentration of Na^+ (30–70 mEq/l) and Cl^- (30–70mEq/l)
- a high concentration of K^+ (up to 5mEq/l), lactate (4–40mEq/l), urea, ammonia and some amino acids.

Only small quantities of toxic substances are lost.

Sweating may also occur in response to emotion and after eating spicy food. In addition to thermoregulation, sweat also helps to maintain the hydration of the horny layer and improves grip on the palms and soles.

Physiology

- Basal cell replication rate: once every 200–400 hours.
- Trans-epidermal cycle time: about 28 days.
- Growth rate for scalp hair: 0.4mm/24h.
- Normal hair fall (scalp): 50–100/24h.
- Fingernail growth: 0.1mm/24h (toenail is less).
- Skin blood flow is controlled by shunting at arteriovenous anastomoses.
- Minimum insensitive perspiration: 0.5 l/24h.

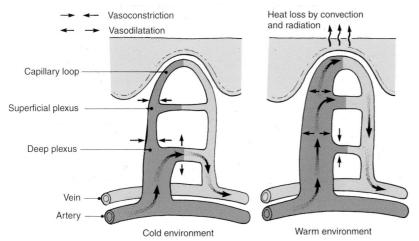

→ ← Vasoconstriction
← → Vasodilatation

Heat loss by convection and radiation

Capillary loop

Superficial plexus

Deep plexus

Vein

Artery

Cold environment   Warm environment

Fig. 4 **Variations in the blood supply to the skin under cold and warm conditions.**

BIOCHEMISTRY OF THE SKIN

The important molecules synthesized by the skin include keratin, melanin, collagen and glycosaminoglycans.

KERATIN

Keratins are high-molecular-weight polypeptide chains produced by keratinocytes (Fig. 1). They are the major constituent of the stratum corneum, hair and nails. The stratum corneum comprises 65% keratin (along with 10% soluble protein, 10% amino acid, 10% lipid and 5% cell membrane).

Keratin polypeptides are of different molecular weight (e.g. 50, 55, 57 and 67 kDa), and different keratins are found at each level of the epidermis, depending on the stage of differentiation. Epidermal keratin contains less cystine and more glycine than the harder, hair keratin.

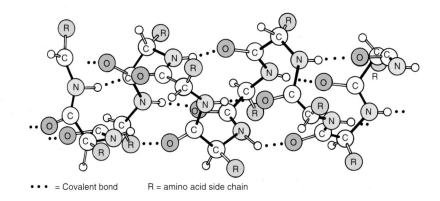

• • • = Covalent bond   R = amino acid side chain

Fig. 1 **Molecular Structure of α-keratin.** The molecule forms a helical coil which if stretched unwinds irreversibly to produce the β form. The covalent bonds linking the cystine molecules provide extra strength.

MELANIN

Melanin is produced from tyrosine (Fig. 2) in melanocytes and takes two forms:

- *eumelanin*, which is more common and gives a brown-black colour
- *phaeomelanin*, which is less common and produces a yellow or red colour.

Most natural melanins are mixtures of eumelanin and phaeomelanin. Melanins act as an energy sink and free-radical scavengers, and absorb the energy of UV radiation.

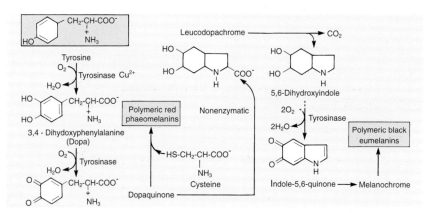

Fig. 2 **Biosynthesis of melanin.** Eumelanin is a high-molecular-weight polymer of complex structure formed by oxidative polymerization. The phaeomelanin polymer is synthesized from dopaquinone and cysteine (via cysteinyl dopa).

COLLAGEN

Collagen is synthesized by fibroblasts (Fig. 3) and is the major structural protein of the dermis, forming 70–80% of its dry weight. The main amino acids in collagen are glycine, proline and hydroxyproline. There are over fourteen types of collagen, at least five of which are found in skin:
- *type I* — found in the reticular dermis
- *type III* — found in the papillary dermis
- *types IV and VII* — found in the basement membrane structures
- *type VIII* — found in endothelial cells.

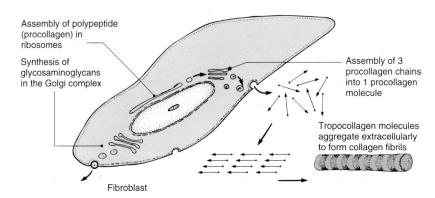

Fig. 3 **Collagen production.** Tropocollagen is formed from three polypeptide chains which are coiled around each other in a triple helix. Assembled collagen fibrils are 100 nm wide, with cross-striations visible with electronmicroscopy every 64 nm.

GLYCOSAMINOGLYCAN (GAG)

The 'ground substance' of skin is largely made up of GAGs, providing viscosity and hydration. In the dermis, chondroitin sulphate is the main GAG, along with dermatan sulphate and hyaluronan.

GAGs often exist as high molecular weight polymers with a protein core. These structures are known as *proteoglycans* (Fig. 4).

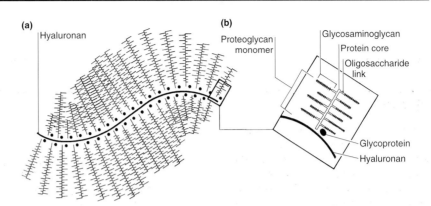

Fig. 4 **Proteoglycan. (a)** Proteoglycan aggregate with central filament of hyaluronan. **(b)** Detailed view of proteoglycan monomer with protein core.

SKIN SURFACE SECRETIONS

The skin surface has a slightly acidic pH (between 6 and 7). Sebum (Table 1), sweat and the horny layer (including intercellular lipid) contribute to the surface conditions, which generally discourage microbial proliferation.

Table 1 **Sebum and epidermal lipid composition**

Component	Sebum (%)	Epidermal lipid (%)
Glyceride/FFA	58	65
Wax esters	26	0
Squalene	12	0
Cholesterol esters	3	15
Cholesterol	1	20

SUBCUTANEOUS FAT

Triglyceride is synthesized from α-glycerophosphate and acyl Co-A. Triglyceride is broken down by lipase to give free fatty acid (FFA) — an energy source — and glycerol (Fig. 5).

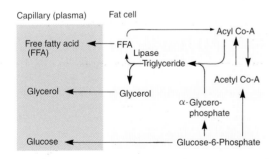

Fig. 5 **Metabolism of subcutaneous fat.**

HORMONES AND THE SKIN
The skin is the site of production of one hormone (Vitamin D), but it is often a target organ for other hormones and is frequently affected in endocrine diseases.

Hormone	Site of production	Effects
Vitamin D	Produced in dermis from precursors though the action of UV radiation	Important for the absorption of calcium and for calcification
Corticosteroids	Adrenal cortex	Receptors on several cells in both epidermis and dermis
		Produce vasoconstriction
		Reduce mitosis by basal cells
		Generate anti-inflammatory effect on leucocytes
		Inhibit phospholipase A
Androgens	Adrenal cortex Gonads	Receptors on hair follicles and sebaceous glands
		Stimulate terminal hair growth and increased output of sebum
Melanocyte-stimulating hormone (MSH) Adrenocorticotrophic hormone (ACTH)	Pituitary gland	Stimulate melanogenesis
Oestrogens	Adrenal Cortex Ovaries	Stimulate melanogenesis
Epidermal growth factor (EGF)	Skin (probably produced at several sites in, as well as outside, the skin)	Receptors found on keratinocytes, hair follicles, sebaceous glands and sweat duct cells
		Stimulates differentiation
		Alters calcium metabolism
Cytokines and eicosanoids	Cell membrane (may be produced by several skin cells, including keratinocytes and lymphocytes)	Effects on immune function, inflammation and cell proliferation

Biochemistry

- Keratins are made up of polypeptide helical coils linked by covalent bonds. They form the horny layer, nails and hair.
- Melanin is a complex polymer synthesized from tyrosine. There are eu- and phaeo- types.
- Collagen is a polypeptide polymer which comprises 75% of the dry weight of the dermis.
- GAG makes up the ground substance of skin.
- Vitamin D: cutaneous UV activation produces active forms.
- Androgen receptors in hair/sebaceous glands make these structures sensitive to the androgen surge of puberty.

IMMUNOLOGY OF THE SKIN

The skin is an important immunological organ and normally contains nearly all the elements of cellular immunity, with the exception of B cells. Much of the original research into immunology was done using the skin as a model.

IMMUNOLOGICAL COMPONENTS OF SKIN

The immunological components of skin can be separated into structures, cells, functional systems and immunogenetics.

STRUCTURES

The epidermal barrier is an important example of innate immunity, since most microorganisms that have contact with the skin do not penetrate it. Equally, the generous blood and lymphatic supplies to the dermis are important channels through which immune cells can pass to or from their sites of action.

CELLS

Langerhans cell
The Langerhans cells of the epidermis are the outermost sentinels of the cellular immune system (Fig. 1). They are dendritic, bone-marrow-derived cells characterized ultrastructurally by a unique cytoplasmic organelle known as the *Birbeck granule*. Langerhans cells play an important role in antigen presentation. Dendritic cells are also seen in the dermis; these lack the Birbeck granule but their other characteristics suggest that they too can present antigen.

T lymphocyte
T lymphocytes are now believed to circulate through normal skin where

they are thought to 'mature'. Different types of T cell are recognized, for example:

- *helper* (facilitate immune reactions)
- *delayed hypersensitivity* (specifically sensitized)
- *cytotoxic*
- *suppressor* (regulate other lymphocytes).

Surface receptors, detectable by the use of monoclonal antibodies on tissue sections, help to categorize the subgroups. Helper T cells often show the CD 4 receptor, and suppressor T cells, the CD 8, though this is not invariable. B lymphocytes are not found in normal skin, but are seen in some disease states.

Mast cell
Mast cells are normal residents of the dermis, as are macrophages. Both may be recruited to the site during inflammatory reactions.

Keratinocyte
Keratinocytes have recently been recognized to have an immunological function. They can produce pro-inflammatory cytokines (especially interleukin-1) and can express on their surface immune reactive molecules such as MHC class II antigens (e.g. HLA-DR) and intercellular adhesion molecules (notably ICAM-1).

FUNCTIONAL SYSTEMS

Skin-associated lymphoid tissue
The skin, with its afferent blood supply, lymphatic drainage, regional lymph nodes, circulating lymphocytes and resident immune cells, can be viewed as forming a regulatory immunological unit.

Cytokines and eicosanoids
Cytokines are soluble molecules that mediate actions between cells. They are produced by T lymphocytes and sometimes by other skin cells, including Langerhans cells, keratinocytes, fibroblasts, endothelial cells and

Table 1 **Some cytokines**

Cytokine	Source	Actions
Gamma interferon	T cells, natural killer cells	HLA-DR & ICAM-1 expression, B cell differentiation
Interleukin-1 (IL-1)	Langerhans cells, T cells, macrophages, keratinocytes, etc.	T cell & macrophage activation, B cell proliferation
IL-2	Activated T cells	T cell cytokine release, B cell proliferation
IL-3	T cells	Pan-specific growth factor

macrophages (Table 1). Eicosanoids are non-specific inflammatory mediators (e.g. prostaglandins, thromboxanes and leukotrienes), and are produced from arachidonic acid by mast cells, macrophages and keratinocytes.

Complement
Activation of the complement cascade down either the classical or the alternative pathways results in molecules that have powerful effects. These include opsonization, lysis, mast-cell degranulation, smooth muscle contraction and chemotaxis for neutrophils and macrophages.

Adhesion molecules
The adhesion molecules, particularly ICAM-1, are cell-surface molecules found on lymphocytes and sometimes on endothelial cells and keratinocytes. By interacting with leucocyte-functional antigens, they help to bind T cells and increase cell trafficking to the area.

IMMUNOGENETICS

The tissue type antigens of an individual are found in the major histocompatibility complex (MHC), located in man on the HLA gene cluster on chromosome 6. The MHC class II antigens, of which the commonest is HLA-DR, are expressed on B lymphocytes, Langerhans cells, some T

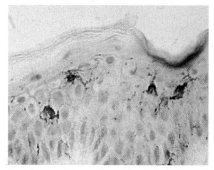

Fig. 1 **Langerhans cell.** The dendritic Langerhans cells form a network in the epidermis. In this section, the Langerhans cells have been stained with a monoclonal antibody to HLA-DR.

cells, macrophages, endothelial cells and keratinocytes (in certain situations). They are vital for immunological recognition, but also are involved in transplant rejection.

In addition, the appearance of specific HLA genes is associated with an increased likelihood of certain diseases, some of which are 'autoimmune' in nature (Table 2).

Table 2 **Skin disease associations of HLA antigens**

Disease	HLA antigen	Frequency (%)	
		Patients	Controls
Psoriasis	B13	21	6
	Bw37	4	2
	Cw23	70	23
Reiter's disease	B27	78	8
Dermatitis herpetiformis	B8	77	25

HYPERSENSITIVITY REACTIONS AND THE SKIN

Hypersensitivity is the term applied when an adaptive immune response is inappropriate or exaggerated to the degree that tissue damage results. The skin can exhibit all the main types of hypersensitivity response.

Type I (immediate)

IgE is bound to the surface of mast cells by Fc receptors. On encountering antigen (e.g. housedust mite, food or pollen) the IgE molecules become crosslinked, producing degranulation and the release of inflammatory mediators. These include preformed mediators (such as histamine) and newly formed ones (e.g. prostaglandins or leukotrienes). The result in the skin is urticaria, although massive histamine release can cause anaphylaxis. The response occurs within minutes, although a delayed component is recognized. Factors other than IgE can cause mast cell degranulation.

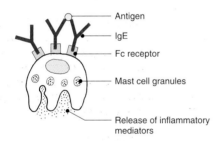

Type II (antibody-dependent cytotoxicity)

Antibodies directed against an antigen on target skin cells or structures induce cytotoxicity by killer T cells or by complement activation. For example, IgG pemphigus antibodies directed against a keratinocyte surface-antigen result in activation of complement, attraction of effector cells and the lysis of the keratinocytes. Intra-epidermal blisters result. Haemolytic anaemia and transfusion reactions are other examples of type II hypersensitivity. Some of these conditions are 'autoimmune'.

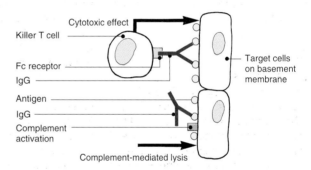

Type III (immune complex disease)

Immune complexes formed by the combination of antigen and antibodies in the blood are deposited in the walls of small vessels, often those of the skin. Complement activation, platelet aggregation and the release of lysosomal enzymes from polymorphs cause vascular damage. This *leucocytoclastic vasculitis* is seen with, for example, systemic lupus erythematosus and dermatomyositis, but also occurs with microbial infections such as infective endocarditis. The 'Arthus reaction' is due to immune complex formation at a local site. It can be induced in the skin by an intradermal injection, and is maximal at 4–10 hours after injection.

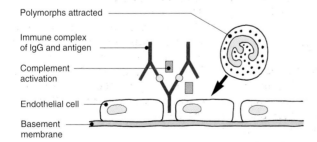

Type IV (cell-mediated or delayed)

Specifically sensitized T lymphocytes have secondary contact with the antigen when it is presented on the surface of antigen-presenting cells (APC). Cytokine release produces T cell activation and amplifies the reaction by recruiting other T cells and macrophages to the site. Tissue damage results which is maximal at 48–72 hours. Allergic contact dermatitis (see p. 30) and the tuberculin reaction to intradermally administered antigen are both forms of type IV reaction. The responses to skin infections such as leprosy or tuberculosis are granulomatous variants of the reaction.

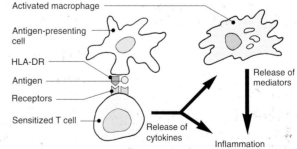
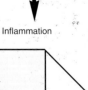

Immunology

- Skin provides a physical barrier to infection.
- Langerhans cells form outposts of the cellular immune system and can present antigens.
- T cells circulate through normal skin and form part of the skin-associated lymphoid tissue.
- Keratinocytes can be immunologically active cells.
- All four types of hypersensitivity reaction occur in the skin.
- Genetic factors modulate immunological responses.

MOLECULAR GENETICS AND THE SKIN

Recent and rapid advances in genetics have had an impact on our understanding of skin diseases. The Human Genome Project hopes to map all human genes by 2005. Genetics has been found to be more complicated than the original Mendelian concept, and common conditions such as atopy occur due to a complex interaction between multiple susceptibility genes and the environment. An average pregnancy carries a 1% risk for a single gene disease and an 0.5% risk for a chromosome disorder but genetically-influenced traits e.g. atopy, are much more common.

THE HUMAN CHROMOSOMES

The human genome comprises 23 pairs of chromosomes which are numbered by size (Fig. 1). Chromosomes are packets of genes with support proteins in a large complex. The karyotype is an individual's number of chromosomes plus their sex chromosome constitution, i.e. 46XX for females and 46XY for males. The phenotype is the expression at a biological level of the genotype, e.g. blue eyes or atopy.

GENES AND DNA

A gene is a segment of deoxyribonucleic acid (DNA) that encodes for ribonucleic acid (RNA) which is translated into a protein. A DNA molecule is composed of multiple variable subunits of 4 nucleotides (2 pyrimidines and 2 purines) on a pentose-phosphate support structure. The bases pair in a consistent way: cytosine with guanine and thymine with adenine. The two DNA strands of the double helix are linked by hydrogen bonds between the complementary base pairs. RNA copies are made and the order of the bases determines the amino acid content of the final protein.

The human genome contains about 80,000 genes. So far, about 15,000 have been located. The mapping of

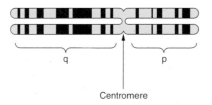

Fig. 1 **Chromosome 2,** divided by the centromere into the shorter (p) and the longer (q) arms, showing banding with the Giemsa stain.

disease-associated genes is often based on observing when two genes adjacent on a chromosome are inherited together (linkage) and using probes to identify markers, preferably in several members of an affected family.

MOLECULAR METHODS

In the laboratory, DNA can be cut by restriction enzymes at specific sites, and DNA segments can be multiplied many times by the polymerase chain reaction (PCR). Fragments of DNA can be identified according to size by gel electrophoresis (Fig. 2). Variations in the DNA sequence for a gene are called polymorphisms and are present in 2% of a stable population. Molecular techniques can be used to:

- detect small amounts of DNA, e.g. of human papilloma virus within a skin cancer
- amplify DNA from a 'candidate' section of an individual's chromosome and compare the base sequences with family members similarly affected by a disorder, thus mapping a specific gene polymorphism characteristic for that disease (Table 1).

Table 1 **Skin conditions or characteristics with definite or probable gene localities on the chromosomes**

Chromosome	Disease or characteristic
1	porphyria cutanea tarda: enzyme (p. 43)
2	Ehlers-Danlos syndrome: collagen III (p. 89)
3	dystrophic epidermolysis bullosa: collagen VII (p. 87)
4	red hair colour
9	familial malignant melanoma (p. 94)
9	xeroderma pigmentosum (p. 89)
9	tuberous sclerosis (p. 88)
11	atopy: asthma and rhinitis (p. 32)
12	epidermolysis bullosa simplex: keratin 2 (p. 87)
12	Darier's disease (p. 87)
14	variegate porphyria: enzyme (p. 43)
15	oculocutaneous albinism (p. 70)
17	neurofibromatosis NF1 (p. 88)
17	Ehlers-Danlos syndrome: collagen I (p. 89)
19	green/blue eye colour
19	brown hair colour
21	Down's syndrome (p. 89)
X	incontinentia pigmenti (p. 89)
X	X-linked ichthyosis: steroid sulphatase

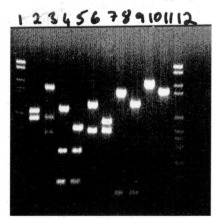

Fig. 2 **Agarose gel electrophoresis** showing migration of DNA after cutting with enzymes, screening for mutations in a keratin gene.

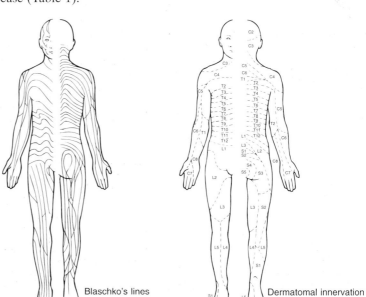

Blaschko's lines   Dermatomal innervation

Fig. 3 **Blaschko's lines** (left) represent the growth trends of embryonic tissue, whereas the **dermatomes** (right) map out areas of skin innervation.

FORMS OF INHERITANCE

An individual with two different genes (alleles) at a particular locus is heterozygous and one who has identical alleles is homozygous. Genes borne on chromosomes other than X and Y are autosomal whereas those on X and Y are sex-linked. Factors governing genetic penetrance are unclear. Heredity is complex and more than simply dominant or recessive:

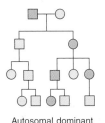
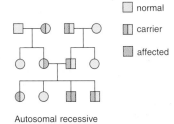

□ normal

◫ carrier

■ affected

Autosomal dominant   Autosomal recessive

Fig. 4 **Autosomal dominant** (left) and **recessive** (right) patterns of inheritance. ○ = females and □= males.

- *Dominant:* Affected individuals (both sexes) are heterozygous for the gene, will have an affected parent (except for new mutations) and have a 50% chance of passing it to their children (Fig. 4).
- *Recessive:* An affected individual (either sex) is homozygous for the gene and both parents will be carriers and healthy. Consanguinity increases the risk. Recessive disorders are often severe. There is a 25% chance of heterozygotes passing the gene to the next generation.
- *X-linked recessive*: Only affects males, as females are healthy carriers.
- *X-linked dominant*: Affects males and females, although some disorders, e.g. incontinentia pigmenti, are lethal in males.

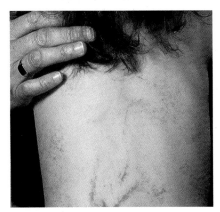

Fig. 5 **Incontinentia pigmenti** showing streaks and whorls that follow the lines of Blaschko.

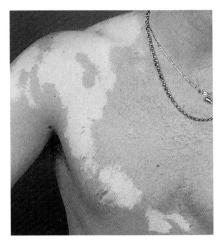

Fig. 6 **Segmental vitiligo;** rather than follow Blaschko's lines this occurs in a dermatomal distribution, suggesting a relationship to skin innervation.

- *Mosaicism:* In mosaicism, an individual has two or more genetically different cell lines. The somatic (post-conceptional) mutation of a single cell in an embryo results in a clone of subtly distinct cells. In the skin, this is revealed by the developmental growth pattern of Blaschko's lines (Fig. 3). Certain dermatoses e.g. naevi and incontinentia pigmenti (Fig. 5) follow these lines, resulting in streaky or whorled patterns where the abnormal clone meets normal cells. A dermatomal distribution (Fig. 6) suggests nerve involvement.
- *Imprinting:* Imprinting involves the differential switching off of genes according to whether they have come from the father or the mother. It may be caused by methylation of DNA.

INHERITANCE OF SPECIFIC SKIN DISORDERS

In psoriasis (p. 26) and atopic eczema (p. 32) a family history is common but the exact mode of inheritance is unclear. Psoriasis may be inherited polygenically or by an autosomal dominant gene with incomplete penetrance. Paternal heredity seems more important than maternal. In contrast, in atopic eczema maternal genes may have a predominant effect. An atopy gene is located on chromosome 11. Inheritance patterns in the rarer con-

ditions are often clearer (Table 2). Epidermolysis bullosa simplex and dystrophica (p. 87), the porphyrias (p. 43), the Ehlers-Danlos syndromes (p. 89) and some other conditions may be dominantly or recessively inherited.

Some dermatoses are associated with polymorphisms in the HLA complex on chromosome 6 (p. 10). These tend to show polygenic inheritance and an association with autoimmunity.

GENE THERAPY

Antenatal diagnosis is possible in certain genodermatoses (p. 87). Recessive disorders in which there is a single gene defect, e.g. steroid sulphatase deficiency in X-linked ichthyosis or recessive epidermolysis bullosa due to a defect in collagen VII, offer scope for genetic treatment. Keratinocytes and fibroblasts are easily cultured and a normal gene can be inserted into the cellular DNA. It remains to be seen whether this will work in practice.

Table 2 **The inheritance of selected skin disorders**

Inheritance	Disorder
Autosomal dominant	Darier's disease (p. 87)
	Dysplastic naevus syndrome (p. 95)
	Ichthyosis vulgaris (p. 86)
	Neurofibromatosis NF1 (p. 88)
	Palmoplantar keratoderma (p. 86)
	Peutz-Jeghers syndrome (p. 71)
	Tuberous sclerosis (p. 88)
Autosomal recessive	Acrodermatitis enteropathica (p. 81)
	Non-bullous ichthyosiform erythroderma (p. 41)
	Phenylketonuria (p. 70)
	Pseudoxanthoma elasticum (p. 89)
	Xeroderma pigmentosum (p. 89)
X-linked recessive	X-linked ichthyosis (p. 86)
X-linked dominant	Incontinentia pigmenti (p. 89)

Molecular genetics and the skin

- The human genome of 23 chromosomes (karyotype 46XY or 46XX) contains 80, 000 genes of which 15, 000 have been located.
- DNA segments can be amplified by PCR and demonstrated by gel electrophoresis.
- The chromosomal location of the marker gene has been mapped for several skin diseases.
- Dominant, recessive and X-linked inheritances are seen but in several disorders heredity is still unclear.
- A dermatosis caused by mosaicism, due to mutation producing more than one cell line, may appear in Blaschko's lines.
- Gene therapy should be possible for some recessive single gene disorders.

BASIC PRINCIPLES

TERMINOLOGY OF SKIN LESIONS

Dermatology has a vocabulary that is quite distinct from other medical specialities and without which it is impossible to describe skin disorders. A *lesion* is a general term for an area of disease, usually small. An *eruption* (or *rash*) is a more widespread skin involvement, normally composed of several lesions which may be the primary pathology (e.g. papules, vesicles or pustules) or due to secondary factors such as scratching or infection (e.g. crusting, lichenification or ulceration).

Below is a selection of other commonly encountered dermatological terms.

MACULE

A macule is a localized area of colour or textural change in the skin. Macules can be hypopigmented, as in vitiligo; pigmented, as in a freckle (**a**); or erythematous as in a capillary haemangioma (**b**).

PAPULE

A papule is a small solid elevation of the skin, generally defined as less than 5 mm in diameter. Papules may be flat-topped, as in lichen planus; dome-shaped, as in xanthomas; or spicular if related to hair follicles.

NODULE

Similar to a papule but larger (i.e. greater than 5 mm in diameter), nodules can involve any layer of the skin and can be oedematous or solid. Examples include a dermatofibroma (below) and secondary deposits.

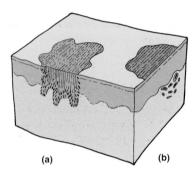

(a)   (b)

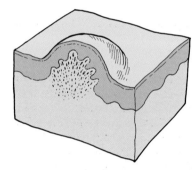

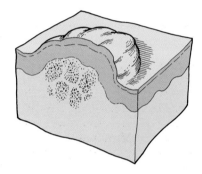

BULLA

A bulla is similar to a vesicle but larger: greater than 5 mm in diameter. The blisters of bullous pemphigoid (**a**) and pemphigus vulgaris (p. 74) are examples.

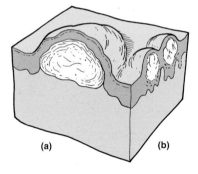

(a)   (b)

VESICLE

A vesicle is a small blister (less than 5 mm in diameter) consisting of clear fluid accumulated within or below the epidermis. Vesicles may be grouped as in dermatitis herpetiformis (sub-epidermal). Intra-epidermal vesicles are shown in the Figure left (**b**).

GLOSSARY OF OTHER DERMATOLOGICAL TERMS

Abscess: A localized collection of pus formed by necrosis of tissue.

Alopecia: Absence of hair from a normally hairy area.

Atrophy: Loss of epidermis, dermis or both. Atrophic skin is thin, translucent and wrinkled with easily visible blood vessels.

Burrow: A tunnel in the skin caused by a parasite, particularly the acarus of scabies.

Callus: Local hyperplasia of the horny layer, often of the palm or sole, due to pressure.

Carbuncle: A collection of boils (furuncles) causing necrosis in the skin and subcutaneous tissues.

Cellulitis: A purulent inflammation of the skin and subcutaneous tissue.

Comedo: A plug of sebum and keratin in the dilated orifice of a pilosebaceous gland.

Crust: Dried exudate (normally serum, blood or pus) on the skin surface.

Ecchymosis: A macular red or purple haemorrhage, more than 2 mm in diameter, in the skin or mucous membrane.

Erosion: A superficial break in the epidermis, not extending into the dermis, which heals without scarring.

Erythema: Redness of the skin due to vascular dilatation.

Excoriation: A superficial abrasion, often linear, which is due to scratching.

Fissure: A linear split in the epidermis, often just extending into the dermis.

PUSTULE

A pustule is a visible collection of free pus in a blister. Pustules may indicate infection (e.g. a furuncle), but not always, as pustules seen in psoriasis, for example, are not infected.

CYST

A cyst is a nodule consisting of an epithelial-lined cavity filled with fluid or semi-solid material. An epidermal ('sebaceous') cyst is shown below.

WHEAL

A wheal is a transitory, compressible papule or plaque of dermal oedema, red or white in colour and usually signifying urticaria.

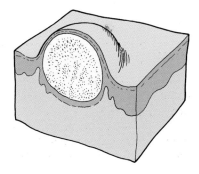 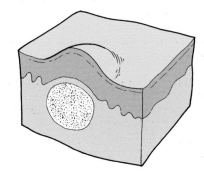 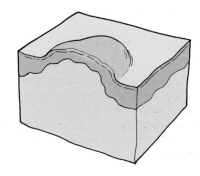

PLAQUE

A plaque is a palpable, plateau-like elevation of skin, usually more than 2cm in diameter. Plaques are rarely more than 5mm in height and can be considered as extended papules. Certain lesions of psoriasis (below) and mycosis fungoides are good examples.

SCALE

A scale is an accumulation of thickened, horny layer keratin in the form of readily detached fragments. Scales usually indicate inflammatory change and thickening of the epidermis. They may be fine, as in 'pityriasis'; white and silvery, as in psoriasis (below); or large and fish-like, as seen in ichthyosis.

ULCER

An ulcer is a circumscribed area of skin loss extending through the epidermis into the dermis. Ulcers are usually the result of impairment of the vascular or nutrient supply to the skin, e.g. due to peripheral arterial disease.

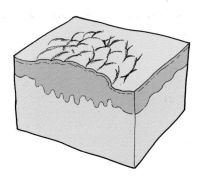 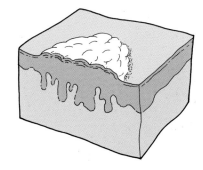 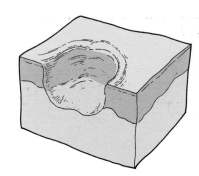

Folliculitis: An inflammation of the hair follicles.
Freckle: A macular area in which there is increased pigment formation by melanocytes.
Furuncle: A pyogenic infection localized in a hair follicle.
Hirsuties: Excessive male-pattern hair growth.
Hypertrichosis: Excessive hair growth in a non-androgenic pattern.
Keloid: An elevated and progressive scar not showing regression.
Keratosis: A horn-like thickening of the skin.
Lichenification: Chronic thickening of the skin with increased skin markings, a result of rubbing or scratching.
Milium: A small white cyst containing keratin.
Papilloma: A nipple-like projection from the skin surface.
Petechia: A haemorrhagic punctuate spot measuring 1–2mm in diameter.
Poikiloderma: A combination of hyperpigmentation, telangiectasia and atrophy seen together in a dermatosis.
Purpura: Extravasation of blood resulting in red discoloration of the skin or mucous membranes.
Scar: The replacement of normal tissue by fibrous connective tissue at the site of an injury.
Stria: An atrophic linear band in the skin — white, pink or purple in colour. The result of connective tissue changes.
Telangiectasia: Dilated dermal blood vessels giving rise to a visible lesion.

TAKING A HISTORY

The truism that 'there is no substitute for a good history' is just as applicable in dermatology as in any other branch of medicine. The time needed to take a history depends on the complaint. For example, the history in a patient with hand warts can usually be completed quickly, but more time and detailed questioning is required for the patient with generalized itching.

History-taking in dermatology can be divided into four basic investigations: the presenting complaint, past medical history, social and family history, and drug history.

PRESENTING COMPLAINT

Prior to any diagnosis, it is essential to find out when, where and how the problem started, what the initial lesions looked like and how they evolved and extended. Symptoms, particularly itching, must be recorded along with any aggravating or exacerbating factors, such as sunlight.

CASE HISTORY 1

An 18-year-old male bank clerk developed a scaly erythematous plaque on the left elbow (Fig. 1) six months ago. It spread to involve the other elbow and both knees, but was not itchy. He developed scaliness in the scalp and nail dystrophy. His mother once had a similar rash.

Diagnosis: psoriasis (p. 26).

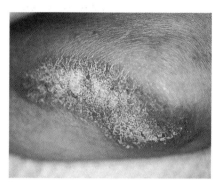

Fig. 1 **Psoriatic plaque on elbow.**

PAST MEDICAL HISTORY

Patients must be asked about any previous skin disease or atopic symptoms, such as hay fever, asthma or childhood eczema. Internal medical disorders may be relevant; these can involve the skin directly or may be associated with certain skin diseases. Prescribed drugs may also cause an eruption.

CASE HISTORY 2

A 29-year-old woman was referred from the department of respiratory medicine where she had recently been diagnosed as having pulmonary sarcoidosis. Three weeks previously she had developed tender, warm erythematous nodules (Fig. 2) on the shins. She was on no medication. An incisional biopsy was performed.

Diagnosis: erythema nodosum (p. 79).

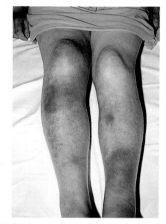

Fig. 2 **Erythema nodosum on the lower legs.**

SOCIAL HISTORY

Many social factors can cause or influence a patient's skin complaint. Occupational factors can induce contact dermatitis or other skin changes, and it is often necessary to ask the patient to explain exactly what he or she does. If the eruption improves when the patient is away from work, occupational factors should be suspected. Hobbies also may involve contact with objects or chemicals that produce contact dermatitis.

A knowledge of the patient's living conditions and home background can also be helpful in understanding a problem and deciding on a treatment. Alcohol intake should be noted (especially if the use of potentially hepatotoxic drugs is being considered), as well as other factors. Living or travelling in warm climates potentially exposes an individual to a wide range of tropical and subtropical infections, and also to strong sunlight.

CASE HISTORY 3

A 45-year-old male printer engineer gave a 6 month history of hand dermatitis (Fig. 3). A few months previously he had started to use the solvent trichloroethylene in his job. Patch testing was negative. On substituting a different solvent the eruption was cleared.

Diagnosis: irritant contact dermatitis (p. 31).

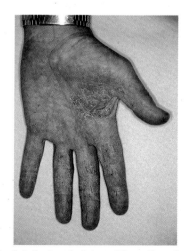

Fig. 3 **Irritant contact dermatitis on the palm of the hand.**

FAMILY HISTORY

A full family history is essential. Some disorders with prominent skin signs are genetically inherited, for example tuberous sclerosis. Others such as psoriasis or atopic eczema have a strong hereditary component. In addition to genetic syndromes, a family history may reveal that other family members have had a recent onset of an eruption similar to that of the patient, suggesting an infection or infestation. It is sometimes also necessary to enquire about sexual contacts.

CASE HISTORY 4

A 25-year-old female shop assistant complained of brownish macules over her back (Fig. 4) and chest which had first appeared in childhood and had gradually increased in number and size. During her teens, she had developed several soft pinkish, painless nodules on the trunk, some of which had become pedunculated. Her father had developed a few similar nodules in later life, and one of her two brothers had brown patches on his skin.

Diagnosis: von Recklinghausen's neurofibromatosis (p. 88).

CASE HISTORY 5

A 15-year-old school boy gave a three-month history of an intensely itchy papular eruption affecting the hands, wrists and penis (Table 1). Several lesions were excoriated (Fig. 5). Treatment with a potent topical steroid was of little benefit. His mother and sister had also recently developed itchy lesions. Close examination showed burrows in the skin.

Diagnosis: scabies (p. 59).

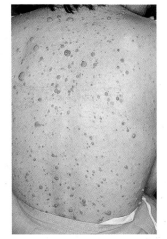

Fig. 4 **Multiple neurofibromas on the back.**

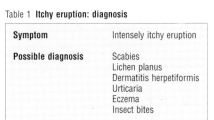

Table 1 **Itchy eruption: diagnosis**

Symptom	Intensely itchy eruption
Possible diagnosis	Scabies
	Lichen planus
	Dermatitis herpetiformis
	Urticaria
	Eczema
	Insect bites

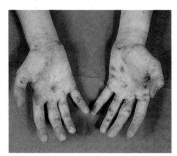

Fig. 5 **Excoriated lesions of scabies.**

DRUG HISTORY

Both prescribed and self-administered medicaments can result in a 'drug eruption'. Almost all patients try an over-the-counter topical preparation (or a friend or relative's ointment) on rashes, and many have had a variety of treatments prescribed which may be inappropriate or may cause irritant or allergic reactions. It is important to quiz the patient about all medicament use, including use of over-the-counter tablets or creams which the patient may well not think relevant.

Cosmetics and moisturizing creams can also cause dermatitis and it is often necessary to ask specifically about their use.

CASE HISTORY 6

A 68-year-old woman had a minor irritating eruption on her forehead. She applied an antihistamine-containing cream which she bought in a chemists. Within 24 hours of applying it, her face became severely swollen (Fig. 6). Patch testing carried out later showed an allergic reaction to the cream.

Diagnosis: medicament dermatitis (p. 31).

CASE HISTORY 7

An 18-year-old female secretary was given griseofulvin for a fungal infection. She went sun-bathing and 12 hours later developed an eruption with a distribution in light-exposed areas (Fig. 7).

Diagnosis: phototoxic drug eruption (p. 43).

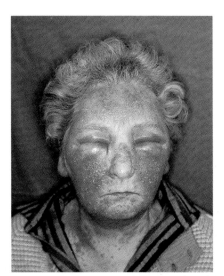

Fig. 6 **Acute allergic contact dermatitis to a topical antihistamine cream.**

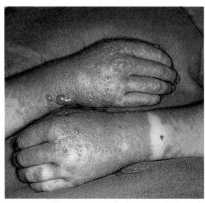

Fig. 7 **Acute phototoxic drug eruption.**

Taking a history

- Elicit the nature and course of the eruption or lesion.
- Identify any factors in the social or family history that may be relevant.
- Record the recent use of any drugs and medications.

EXAMINING THE SKIN

The skin needs to be examined in good, preferably natural, light. The whole of the skin should be examined, ideally; this is essential for atypical or widespread eruptions (Fig. 1). Looking at the whole skin often reveals diagnostic lesions that the patient is unaware of or may think unimportant. In the elderly, thorough skin examination often allows the early detection of unexpected but treatable malignant conditions.

Skin examination is difficult for the non-dermatologist, and the novice needs a pattern to follow. It is important to:

- note the distribution and colour of the lesions
- examine the morphology of individual lesions, their size, shape, border changes and spatial relationship. Palpation reveals the consistency of a lesion
- assess the nails, hair and mucous membranes, sometimes in combination with a general examination (e.g. for lymphadenopathy)
- utilize special techniques, e.g. microscopy of scrapings or the use of Wood's light, where applicable.

DISTRIBUTION

Stand back from the patient and observe the pattern of the eruption (Fig. 1). Determine whether it is localized (e.g. a tumour) or widespread (e.g. a rash). If the latter, determine if the eruption is symmetrical and, if so, peripheral or central. Note whether it involves the flexures (e.g. atopic eczema) or the extensor aspects (e.g.

psoriasis). Is it limited to sun-exposed areas? Is it linear?

Dermatomal patterns are also seen. Herpes zoster (shingles) is the commonest example of this, but some naevi also appear in this guise or follows Blaschko's lines (p. 12). Regional patterns (Fig. 1), e.g. involvement of the groin or axilla, will

suggest certain diagnoses to the experienced physician. For example, guttate psoriasis and tinea versicolor tend to occur on the trunk, whereas lichen planus often occurs around the wrists, and contact dermatitis frequently affects the face or hands.

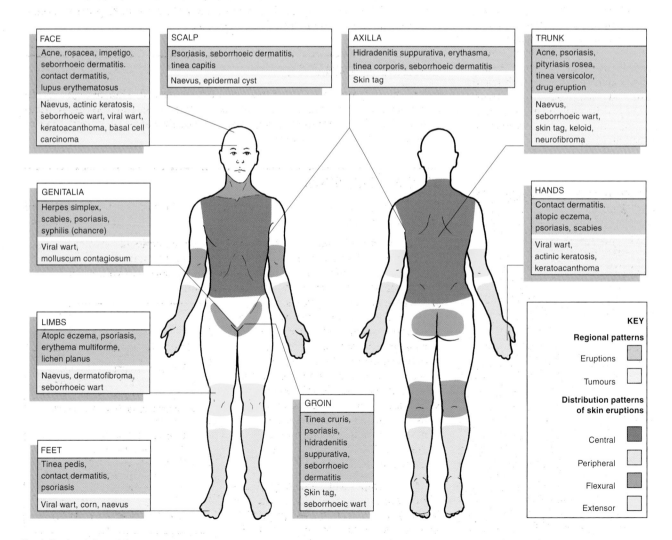

FACE
Acne, rosacea, impetigo, seborrhoeic dermatitis, contact dermatitis, lupus erythematosus

Naevus, actinic keratosis, seborrhoeic wart, viral wart, keratoacanthoma, basal cell carcinoma

SCALP
Psoriasis, seborrhoeic dermatitis, tinea capitis

Naevus, epidermal cyst

AXILLA
Hidradenitis suppurativa, erythasma, tinea corporis, seborrhoeic dermatitis

Skin tag

TRUNK
Acne, psoriasis, pityriasis rosea, tinea versicolor, drug eruption

Naevus, seborrhoeic wart, skin tag, keloid, neurofibroma

GENITALIA
Herpes simplex, scabies, psoriasis, syphilis (chancre)

Viral wart, molluscum contagiosum

HANDS
Contact dermatitis, atopic eczema, psoriasis, scabies

Viral wart, actinic keratosis, keratoacanthoma

LIMBS
Atoplc eczema, psoriasis, erythema multiforme, lichen planus

Naevus, dermatofibroma, seborrhoeic wart

GROIN
Tinea cruris, psoriasis, hidradenitis suppurativa, seborrhoeic dermatitis

Skin tag, seborrhoeic wart

FEET
Tinea pedis, contact dermatitis, psoriasis

Viral wart, corn, naevus

KEY
Regional patterns
Eruptions
Tumours
Distribution patterns of skin eruptions
Central
Peripheral
Flexural
Extensor

Fig. 1 **Regional dermatology.**

CASE HISTORY 1

An 8-year-old girl gave a 12-month history of an itchy eruption affecting the antecubital and popliteal fossae (Fig. 2). Her mother had a similar rash as a child. The pattern and the morphology were characteristic.

Diagnosis: atopic eczema (p. 32).

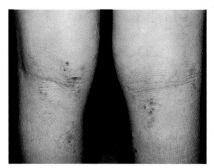

Fig. 2 **Atopic eczema affecting the popliteal fossae.**

CASE HISTORY 2

Six weeks ago an 18-year-old girl developed a slightly itchy linear area running down the medial aspect of her right leg (Fig. 3). Dermatological conditions giving a linear eruption include lichen planus, morphoea, psoriasis and linear epidermal naevus.

Diagnosis: lichen striatus, a self-limiting inflammatory dermatitis of unknown origin.

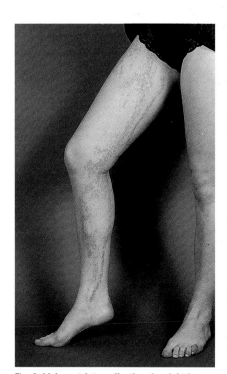

Fig. 3 **Lichen striatus affecting the right leg.**

INDIVIDUAL LESION MORPHOLOGY

A hand lens is often helpful in looking at individual lesions. Palpation (often neglected by medical students) is also important to determine the consistency, depth and texture. Definitions of lesions are given on page 14.

Lesions may be monomorphic (e.g. guttate psoriasis) or pleomorphic (e.g. chickenpox). There may also be secondary changes on top of primary lesions. The local configuration of lesions is often of diagnostic help (Table 1). Determine whether the lesions are grouped, linear or annular, or if they show the Koebner phenomenon (p. 26) whereby lesions appear in an area of trauma which is often linear, e.g. a scratch.

Table 1 **Configuration of lesions**

Configuration	Condition
Linear	Psoriasis, lichen striatus, linear epidermal naevus, lichen planus, morphoea
Grouped	Dermatitis herpetiformis, insect bites, herpes simplex
Annular	Tinea corporis (ringworm), mycosis fungoides, urticaria, granuloma annulare, annular erythemas
Koebner phenomenon	Lichen planus, psoriasis, viral warts, molluscum contagiosum, sarcoidosis

NAILS, HAIR AND MUCOUS MEMBRANES

The nails, scalp and hair frequently show diagnostic and even pathognomonic signs (p. 64). With any unusual or atypical eruption, the mucous membranes of the mouth and genitalia may show important changes, such as the oral involvement by Wickham's striae in lichen planus, the oral lesions in Kaposi's sarcoma, or the vulval involvement with lichen sclerosus.

GENERAL EXAMINATION

Palpation of lymph nodes is important in patients with skin malignancy. In patients with a skin lymphoma, a full examination is needed, looking particularly for lymphadenopathy and hepatosplenomegaly. Palpation of pedal pulses is vital in patients with leg ulcers.

SPECIAL TECHNIQUES

Clinical diagnoses of many skin conditions can be verified by a number of special techniques.

- **Ultraviolet radiation.** Use of Wood's lamp, which emits ultraviolet radiation, will cause hair and, to a lesser extent, the skin to fluoresce in certain fungal infections. It may also be used to show up vitiligo, or hypopigmented macules in tuberous sclerosis.
- **Microscopy.** Viewing skin scrapings (treated with a potassium hydroxide solution) under a light microscope can be helpful in confirming the presence of fungal hyphae. In scabies, the acarus can be extracted using a needle and viewed under the microscope.
- **Surgical biopsy.** Surgery can be used either to excise lesions as a treatment (and to confirm the diagnosis) or to help make the diagnosis.

Other important ancillary techniques are photography (to record the lesions), patch testing (see page 118) and prick tests for type I (IgE-mediated) hypersensitivity.

Examining the skin

- Examine the entire skin surface.
- Use a hand lens and adequate illumination.
- Gently palpate lesions to assess texture.
- Look at the nails, hair and mucous membranes.
- Observe for distribution, individual lesion morphology and configuration.
- Always microscope scrapings if a fungal infection is a possibility.

BASICS OF MEDICAL THERAPY

The treatment of skin disease includes topical, systemic, intralesional, radiation and surgical modalities. Specific treatments are detailed in Sections II and III; below is an overview of dermatological therapies.

TOPICAL THERAPY

Topical treatment has the advantage of direct delivery and reduced systemic toxicity. It consists of a *vehicle* or base which often contains an active ingredient (Table 1).

Vehicles are defined as follows:

- **Lotion**. A liquid vehicle, often aqueous or alcohol-based, which may contain a salt in solution. A *shake lotion* contains an insoluble powder (e.g. calamine lotion).
- **Cream**. A semi-solid emulsion of oil-in-water; contains an emulsifier for stability, and a preservative to prevent overgrowth of micro-organisms.
- **Gel**. A transparent semi-solid, non-greasy emulsion.
- **Ointment**. A semi-solid grease or oil, containing little or no water but sometimes with added powder. No preservative is usually needed. The active ingredient is suspended rather than dissolved.
- **Paste**. An ointment base with a high proportion of powder (starch or zinc oxide) producing a stiff consistency.

THERAPEUTIC PROPERTIES OF THE VEHICLE

Lotions evaporate and cool the skin and are useful for inflamed/exudative conditions, e.g. for wet wraps (p. 33). The high water content of a cream means that it mostly evaporates; it is also non-greasy and easy to apply or remove. Ointments are best for dry skin conditions such as eczema. They rehydrate and occlude, but (being greasy) are difficult to wash off and are less acceptable to patients than creams. Pastes are ideal for applying to well-defined surfaces, such as psoriatic plaques, but are also hard to remove.

QUANTITIES REQUIRED

One application to the whole body requires 20-30 g of ointment. The adult face or neck requires 1 g, trunk (each side) 3 g, arm $1\frac{1}{2}$ g, hand $\frac{1}{2}$ g, leg 3 g and foot 1 g. A useful guide for patients is the *'fingertip unit'* (FTU) – the amount of cream or ointment that

Table 1 **An overview of topical medicaments**

Drug	Indications	Pharmacology
Corticosteroids	Eczemas, psoriasis, lichen planus, discoid lupus erythematosus, sunburn, pityriasis rosea, mycosis fungoides, photodermatoses, lichen sclerosus	Mode of action is through vasoconstrictive, anti-inflammatory and anti-proliferative effects; medication is available in different strengths; side-effects important
Antiseptics	Skin sepsis, leg ulcers	Amongst the more commonly used are chlorhexidine, silver nitrate, potassium permanganate, and iodine compounds
Antibiotics	Acne, rosacea, folliculitis, impetigo, infected eczema	Chlortetracycline, neomycin, bacitracin, gramicidin, polymixin, sodium fusidate, and mupirocin are available; resistance and sensitization are potential problems. Metronidazole is used for rosacea.
Antifungals	Fungal infections of the skin, *Candida albicans* infections	Nystatin, clotrimazole, miconazole, econazole, terbinafine, ketoconazole, sulconazole and amorolfine are available
Antiviral agents	Herpes simplex, herpes zoster	Idoxuridine, aciclovir
Parasiticidals	Scabies, lice	Benzyl benzoate, lindane, permethrin and malathion for scabies; malathion, permethrin and carbaryl for lice — applied as lotion or shampoo
Coal tar	Psoriasis, eczema	Presumed anti-inflammatory and anti-proliferative effects; available as creams, shampoos and in paste bandages
Dithranol	Psoriasis	Anti-proliferative effects; available as creams, pastes and ointments
Vitamin D analogues	Psoriasis	Calcipotriol and tacalcitol inhibit keratinocyte proliferation and promote differentiation; creams and ointments available
Keratolytics	Acne, scaly eczemas	Salicylic acid, benzoyl peroxide and tretinoin

can be applied to the terminal phalanx of the index finger (Fig. 1). One FTU equals $\frac{1}{2}$ g.

The safe maximum amount varies with the strength of the steroid, the age of the patient and the length of treatment. For 1% hydrocortisone, adults can use 150–200g/week, but children can use only 60 g and babies as little as 20 g. Creams/ointments are applied twice daily except for Elocon, Cutivate and Curatoderm (tacalcitol), which are used once daily.

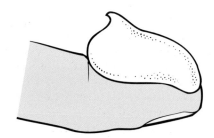

Fig. 1 **The fingertip unit (FTU) = $\frac{1}{2}$ g.**

PHARMACOKINETICS

The ability of a drug to penetrate the epidermis depends on several factors. These include:

- the drug's molecular structure
- the vehicle
- the site on the body (absorption is greatest through the eyelid and scrotum)
- whether or not the skin is diseased.

EMOLLIENTS

Emollients help dry-skin conditions such as eczema and ichthyosis by re-establishing the surface lipid layer and enhancing rehydration of the epidermis. Common emollients include emulsifying ointment, aqueous cream, Unguentum Merck, Diprobase, Hydromol and Aquadrate creams. Oils added to bath water can also help (e.g. Oilatum, Balneum, Alpha-Keri and Emulsiderm).

DRESSINGS AND HOSPITAL ADMISSION

Many departments now have treatment centres where daily dressings and UV treatments are given. If outpatient management is unsuccessful, hospital admission may be needed. Dressings, either for the outpatient or the inpatient, consist of stockinette gauze applied to the trunk or limbs after the ointments have been put on. These must be changed once or twice a day. Leg ulcer dressings may be changed less frequently, depending on the type of application used.

Bandages impregnated with tar are sometimes helpful for leg ulcers and eczema. Many types of paraffin gauze, hydrocolloid and seaweed dressings are now available for leg ulcers.

TOPICAL STEROIDS

A summary of the indications for topical treatment with corticosteroids is given in Table 1. The relative potencies of the more commonly prescribed preparations are shown in Table 2.

Side-effects of topical steroid therapy

The use of topical steroids carries the potential for harmful side-effects. These include:

- atrophy of the skin — thinning, erythema, telangiectasia, purpura and striae (p. 106)
- induction of acne or perioral dermatitis, and exacerbation of rosacea
- atypical fungal infection (tinea incognito); bacterial or viral infections may be potentiated by treatment
- allergic contact dermatitis (due to a component of the preparation or to the steroid)
- systemic absorption — suppression of the pituitary-adrenal axis, Cushingoid appearance, growth retardation
- tachyphylaxis — reduced responsiveness to the steroid after prolonged use.

Table 2 **Relative potencies of topical steroids**

Potency	Example (Generic name)	Proprietary name (UK)
Mild	Hydrocortisone 1% and 2.5%	Efcortelan, Hydrocortistab, Hydrocortisyl
Moderately potent	Clobetasone butyrate 0.05%	Eumovate
	Desoxymethasone 0.05%	Stiedex
	Flurandrenolone 0.0125%	Haelan
	Alclometasone dipropionate 0.05%	Modrasone
Potent	Betamethasone valerate 0.1%	Betnovate (Valisone USA)
	Beclomethasone dipropionate 0.025%	Propaderm
	Betamethasone dipropionate 0.05%	Diprosone (UK and USA)
	Budesonide 0.025%	Preferid
	Fluocinolone acetonide 0.025%	Synalar (UK and USA)
	Fluocinonide 0.05%	Metosyn (Lidex USA)
	Fluticasone propionate 0.05%	Cutivate (UK and USA)
	Hydrocortisone 17-butyrate 0.1%	Locoid (UK and USA)
	Mometasone furoate 0.1%	Elocon
	Triamcinolone acetonide 0.1%	Adcortyl (Aristocort, Kenalog USA)
Very potent	Clobetasol propionate 0.05%	Dermovate (Temovate USA)
	Diflucortolone valerate 0.3%	Nerisone Forte

SYSTEMIC THERAPY

Systemic treatments are used particularly for the more serious conditions and for infections. Details are given in Table 3.

OTHER TREATMENTS

A wide variety of other, more specialized treatments exists for specific skin conditions. Corticosteroids are sometimes injected directly into lesions (e.g. to treat keloids). Certain disorders are responsive to ultraviolet B or photochemotherapy (p. 43).

In the past, X-irradiation was used to treat a variety of skin conditions including psoriasis, acne, tinea capitis, tuberculosis of the skin and hand eczema. There are now very few indications for X-ray treatment of non-malignant disease, although irradiation is of great value in several types of skin tumour.

Cryotherapy, in which liquid nitrogen is applied to the skin, is currently widely used in dermatology (p. 105). It is mainly employed for the treatment of benign or pre-malignant skin tumours.

Table 3 **An overview of systemic therapy**

Group	Drug	Indications
Corticosteroids	Prednisolone usually	Bullous disorders, connective tissue disease, vasculitis
Cytotoxics	Methotrexate	Psoriasis, sarcoidosis
	Hydroxyurea	Psoriasis
	Azathioprine	Bullous disorders, chronic actinic dermatitis
Immunosuppressants	Cyclosporin	Psoriasis, atopic eczema
	Gold	Bullous disorders, lupus erythematosus
Retinoids	Acitretin	Keratinization disorders
	Isotretinoin	Acne
Antifungals	Griseofulvin	Fungal infection
	Ketoconazole	Fungal infection (*C. albicans* too)
	Itraconazole	Fungal infection, candidiasis
	Terbinafine	Fungal infection
Antibiotics	Various	Skin sepsis, acne, rosacea
Antivirals	Aciclovir	Herpes simplex/zoster
	Famciclovir	Herpes zoster, genital herpes simplex
Antihistamines	H1 blockers	Urticaria, eczema
Antiandrogens	Cyproterone	Acne (females only)
Antimalarials	Hydroxychloroquine	Lupus erythematosus, porphyria cutanea tarda
Antileprotic	Dapsone	Dermatitis herpetiformis, leprosy, vasculitis

Basics of medical therapy

- Correct diagnosis is essential to ensure appropriate treatment.
- When using topical steroids:
  - use the lowest potency that is effective
  - look out for side-effects, especially atrophy
  - emollients can help reduce the steroid requirement.
- Explain the treatment to the patient and preferably give a written handout; this helps compliance.
- Use the simplest treatment possible; patients easily get mixed up if they have several different tubes to use.

EPIDEMIOLOGY OF SKIN DISEASE

Skin disease is very common. About 10% of a general practitioner's work load in the UK and 6% of hospital outpatient referrals can be accounted for by skin problems. Skin disease is also economically significant; it is the single most frequent occupational cause of loss of time from work and is the commonest industrial disease (p. 116).

In any discussion of epidemiology it is important to first define the terms used:

- *Prevalence* refers to the proportion of a defined population affected by a disease at any given time.
- *Incidence* is defined as the proportion of a population experiencing the disorder within a stated period of time (usually one year).

The type, prevalence and incidence of skin disease all depend on social, economic, geographic, racial, cultural and age-related factors.

SKIN DISEASE IN THE GENERAL POPULATION

Reliable population statistics are difficult to obtain, but it appears that in the UK the prevalence of skin disease needing some sort of medical care is about 20%. Eczema, acne and infective disorders (including warts) are the commonest complaints (Fig. 1). Only a minority seek medical advice.

SKIN DISEASE IN GENERAL PRACTICE AND HOSPITALS

The *precise* proportion of skin disorders seen in general practice (Fig. 2) will vary with the age structure of the population served, the amount of industry in the area and socio-economic factors.

In the UK, hospital clinics are composed of patients referred from general practitioners, i.e. they are a selected population who have already been treated by at least one doctor (Fig. 3). Referral patterns vary between different regions, depending on local facilities, interests and customs. Within a year, just over 1% of the population is referred for a dermatological opinion. In the mid-1990s, a quarter of all new referrals required a minor surgical procedure.

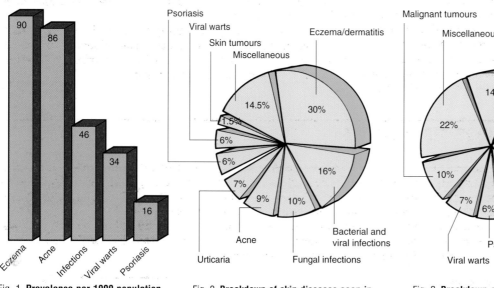

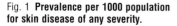

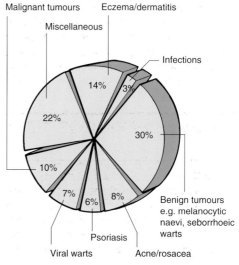

Fig. 1 **Prevalence per 1000 population for skin disease of any severity.**

Fig. 2 **Breakdown of skin diseases seen in general practice (% of total).**

Fig. 3 **Breakdown of skin disease seen in a hospital dermatological clinic (% of total).**

SOCIO-ECONOMIC FACTORS

Improvements in the standard of living resulting from the 19th century industrialization of Britain were accompanied by a fall in the incidences of most infectious diseases and a decline in the infant mortality rate. Better nutrition, improved living conditions and the introduction of hygienic measures are thought to have been important. Most forms of infectious disease, including those of the skin, are now more common in the Third World than in Western countries, and it would seem that the poorer standards of living in these countries are a cause of this.

However, industrialization brings its own problems. Industrial dermatitis is not uncommon in the UK and mild cases are often not reported. Increased sophistication in Western countries also means that patients now want something done about disorders or minor imperfections that would not have bothered past generations.

Changes in social fashion have also brought about changes in skin disease.

For example, the habit of sun bathing which became popular in the 1970s seems to have resulted in an increase in the incidence of malignant melanoma in the 1980s and 1990s.

The media have also had an effect: the numerous articles and programmes on the potential problems associated with a change in pigmented naevi have produced a flood of referrals of worried patients seeking reassurance about their lesions!

GEOGRAPHIC FACTORS

Humid conditions found in hot countries predispose to fungal and bacterial infections, and to other conditions such as 'prickly heat' (an itchy eruption due to blocked sweat ducts). Ultraviolet radiation in sunny climes will obviously result in actinic damage and malignant change in the skin of non-pigmented migrants to the area.

Figure 4 shows a comparison between some common complaints in different geographic locations. The rates for bacterial and fungal infections show variation, and skin cancers are more common in Australia. However, the figures for eczema/ dermatitis are remarkably constant.

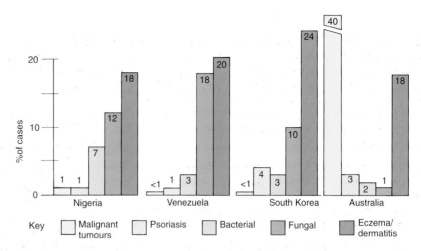

Fig. 4 **Geographic variations in hospital attendances (%) with some common dermatological disorders.**

RACIAL AND CULTURAL FACTORS

Quite apart from the obvious differences in pigmentation, the skin structure varies between the different races (p. 114). For example, hair is often spiral in Africans but straight in mongoloids. In caucasoids, hair is more variable and may be straight, wavy or helical. Skin tumours and actinic damage are seen more in caucasoids than in Africans, with mongoloids showing an intermediate incidence. Keloids and hair problems, such as pseudofolliculitis (p. 115), are more common in Africans, whereas mongoloid skin has a tendency to become lichenified and acne may be less frequent. Vitiligo appears to have a similar incidence in all races, but is more conspicuous in those with a dark skin.

Cultural factors may bring problems. For example, 'hot-combing', practiced by some Afro-Caribbeans, may result in alopecia, while the use of certain traditional oils or cosmetics can produce a dermatitis.

AGE AND SEX PREVALENCE OF DERMATOSES

Different disorders are associated with different times of life (Table 1). Some disorders occur throughout life but are more common at certain ages, whereas others are almost exclusively encountered in defined age-groups. For example, atopic eczema is most common in infants, acne is mainly seen in adolescents and psoriasis has its peak onset in the second and third decades of life. Certain disorders tend to appear in middle age, for example, pemphigus and malignant melanoma. In old age, degenerative and malignant skin conditions are often found. Thus the age structure of the population will influence the type of dermatology practiced.

Some conditions are more common to a specific sex (Table 2).

Table 1 **Age-related onset of selected skin disorders**

Age	Disorder
Childhood	Port-wine stain and strawberry naevi, ichthyosis, erythropoietic protoporphyria, epidermolysis bullosa, atopic eczema, infantile seborrhoeic dermatitis, urticaria pigmentosa, viral exanthems, viral warts, molluscum contagiosum, impetigo
Adolescence	Melanocytic naevi, acne, psoriasis (notably guttate), seborrhoeic dermatitis, vitiligo, pityriasis rosea
Early adulthood	Psoriasis, seborrhoeic dermatitis, lichen planus, dermatitis herpetiformis, lupus erythematosus, vitiligo, tinea versicolor
Middle age	Porphyria cutanea tarda, lichen planus, rosacea, pemphigus vulgaris, venous ulceration, malignant melanoma, basal cell carcinoma, mycosis fungoides
Old age	Asteatotic eczema, 'senile' pruritus, bullous pemphigoid, venous and arterial ulcers, seborrhoeic warts, solar keratosis, solar elastosis, Campbell-de-Morgan spots, basal cell carcinoma, squamous cell carcinoma, herpes zoster

Table 2 **Skin disorders with a male or female preponderance**

Sex	Disorder
Female	Palmoplantar pustulosis, lichen sclerosus, lupus erythematosus, systemic sclerosis, morphoea, rosacea, dermatitis artefacta, venous ulceration, intraepidermal carcinoma, malignant melanoma
Male	Seborrhoeic dermatitis, dermatitis herpetiformis, porphyria cutanea tarda, polyarteritis nodosa, pruritus ani, tinea pedis and cruris, mycosis fungoides, squamous cell carcinoma

Epidemiology

- The commonest skin diseases in the general community are eczema, acne, and infections, including viral warts.
- About 20% of the general population have some sort of skin disorder requiring medical attention.
- Skin disease accounts for 10% of all consultations in general practice.
- Better living conditions reduce skin infection, but excess sun on a white skin predisposes to skin cancer.

BODY IMAGE, THE PSYCHE AND THE SKIN

THE STRESS OF HAVING SKIN DISEASE

The potentially harsh psychological effects of having chronic skin disease tend to be underestimated. Up to 30% of skin outpatients suffer 'psychological distress' from their condition. This is particularly understandable in the teenager with acne, or in someone who has extensive psoriasis or eczema. In both these situations, the individual's devalued body-image may be out of proportion to the objective severity of his or her skin problem. Skin diseases can thus make patients into 'social lepers' who feel that their social lives are restricted because other people do not want to mix with them.

Patients sometimes feel that their disorder is either caused directly by, or exacerbated by, 'stress'. This is difficult to prove, as it is often impossible to differentiate reactive from aetiological states. Many dermatologists believe that psychological factors can, for example, make eczema and psoriasis worse, but most would also agree that these are stressful conditions in their own right. However, it is accepted that there are a small number of conditions that are of psychogenic origin.

SKIN DISORDERS OF PSYCHOGENIC ORIGIN

DERMATITIS ARTEFACTA

Dermatitis artefacta (Fig. 1) should be suspected from the presence of lesions with bizarre shapes (often linear or angular and in accessible sites) which do not conform to natural disease. The lesions are often ulcerated or crusted and do not heal as expected, although they do heal if occluded. Blisters or bruises are also sometimes found.

The condition tends to occur in young women. Confrontation is not recommended, as this may lead to an angry denial. Management is aimed at excluding genuine disease, establishing a rapport with the patient and gently trying to investigate the presence of psychological stresses, for example in the home or work environment, or in social or sexual relationships.

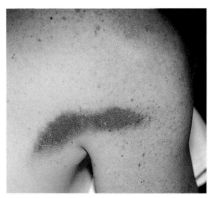

Fig. 1 **Dermatitis artefacta: a linear lesion.**

DELUSIONS OF BODY IMAGE

Patients may present with no objective skin disease but still complain of symptoms such as burning or redness of the face, or display a preoccupation with an imagined problem such as excessive facial hair. This condition, sometimes known as dysmorphophobia, is usually seen in women, although it does occur in men, who may complain of a burning scrotum. Most of these patients are depressed, although some may show signs of schizophrenia. Psychiatric referral is needed for those with true delusions.

DELUSIONS OF PARASITOSIS

Patients with this condition are convinced that their skin is infested with parasites, and they often bring collections of keratin and debris to support their contention. Self-induced excoriation of the skin may be seen. It mainly occurs in women over the age of 40 years. Most patients do not have an organic psychosis, but they are often obsessionals and do have a monosymptomatic hypochondriasis. Treatment is difficult. It is necessary to exclude a true parasitosis. The antipsychotic drug pimozide (in a dose of 2 to 10 mg daily) is helpful in some patients.

TRICHOTILLOMANIA

Rubbing, pulling and twisting the hair is not uncommon in children and results in thinning of scalp hair, which recovers spontaneously. When the condition occurs in adults, the hair may be cut using scissors or a razor, and the prognosis is not so good.

NEUROTIC EXCORIATIONS

Accessible areas of the skin, particularly the forearms and back of the neck, are commonly involved in this condition, with excoriated lesions in a variety of stages of evolution from ulcers to healed scars (Fig. 2). The damage is inflicted as a result of an uncontrollable itch, but there is no primary lesion. Effective occlusion will allow healing. *Acne excoriée* is a variant seen in young women who squeeze and pick their lesions, resulting in artefactual erosions.

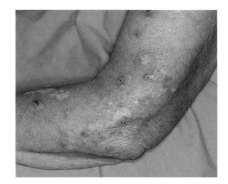

Fig. 2 **Neurotic excoriations on the arm.** Some have healed to leave hypopigmented scars.

Body image, the psyche and the skin

- Psychological stress is common in patients with skin disease.
- Some skin disorders (e.g. eczema and psoriasis) may get worse at times of stress in certain patients.
- A small number of skin diseases are psychogenic in origin.

DISEASES

PSORIASIS — Epidemiology, Pathophysiology and Presentation

DEFINITION

Psoriasis is a chronic, non-infectious inflammatory dermatosis characterized by well-demarcated erythematous plaques topped by silvery scales (Fig. 1).

EPIDEMIOLOGY

Psoriasis affects 2% of the population in Europe and North America, but is less common in Africa and Japan. The sex incidence is equal. The condition may start at any age, even in the elderly, but the peak onset is in the 2nd and 3rd decades. It is unusual in children less than 8 years old.

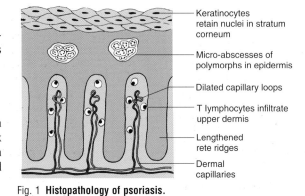

Keratinocytes retain nuclei in stratum corneum

Micro-abscesses of polymorphs in epidermis

Dilated capillary loops

T lymphocytes infiltrate upper dermis

Lengthened rete ridges

Dermal capillaries

Fig. 1 **Histopathology of psoriasis.**

AETIOPATHOGENESIS

Genetics

Inherited polygenic factors predispose to the development of psoriasis. About 35% of patients show a family history, and identical twin studies show a concordance of 80%. There is a 25% probability that a child with one parent who has psoriasis will be similarly affected, but this increases to 60% if both parents have psoriasis. There are strong correlations with the HLA antigens CW6, B13 and B17. Environmental factors are thought to trigger the disease in susceptible individuals.

Epidermal kinetics and metabolism

The epidermal cell proliferation rate is increased 20 fold or more in psoriasis, and the germinative cell population is expanded. The epidermal turnover time is reduced from 28 days to 4 days, although individual cell-cycle times are not much changed. Arachidonic acid metabolites in the epidermis are altered. For example, the level of leukotriene B4 is increased, and this may explain the chemotaxis of polymorphonuclear leucocytes to the psoriatic epidermis.

Precipitating factors

A number of precipitating factors are associated with the disorder:

- *Koebner phenomenon.* Trauma to the epidermis and dermis, such as a scratch or surgical scar (p. 19), can precipitate psoriasis in the damaged skin (see Fig. 2).
- *Infection.* Typically, a streptococcal sore throat may precipitate guttate psoriasis.
- *Drugs.* Beta-blockers, lithium and antimalarials can make psoriasis worse or precipitate it.

- *Sunlight.* Exposure to sunlight can aggravate psoriasis (in about 10%), although in the majority it has a beneficial effect.
- *Psychological stress.* The effects are difficult to assess; some clinicians believe it can exacerbate psoriasis.

PATHOLOGY

The epidermis is thickened, with keratinocytes retaining their nuclei (Fig. 1). There is no granular layer and keratin builds up loosely at the horny layer. The rete ridges are elongated and polymorphs infiltrate up into the stratum corneum where they form micro-abscesses. Capillaries are dilated in the papillary dermis. Lymphocytes are seen infiltrating the earliest psoriatic lesions and may initiate several of the changes observed.

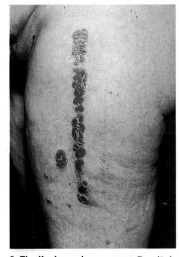

Fig. 2 **The Koebner phenomenon.** Psoriasis has developed in a surgical scar.

CLINICAL PRESENTATION

Psoriasis varies in severity from the trivial to the life-threatening. Its appearance and behaviour also range widely from the readily recognizable chronic plaques on the elbows to the acute generalized pustular form. Psoriasis can be confused with other conditions (see Table 1).

Presentation patterns of psoriasis include:

- plaque
- guttate
- flexural
- localized forms
- generalized pustular
- nail involvement
- erythoderma (p. 40).

Plaque

Well-defined, disc-shaped plaques (Fig. 3) involving the elbows, knees, scalp hair margin or sacrum are the classic presentation (see also p. 16, Fig. 1). The plaques are usually red and covered by waxy white scales which if

Table 1 **Differential diagnosis of psoriasis**

Variant of psoriasis	Differential diagnosis
Plaque psoriasis	Psoriasiform drug eruption (due to beta-blockers)
	Hypertrophic lichen planus
Palmoplantar psoriasis	Hyperkeratotic eczema
	Reiter's disease
Scalp psoriasis	Seborrhoeic dermatitis
Guttate psoriasis	Pityriasis rosea
Flexural psoriasis	Candidiasis of the flexures
Nail psoriasis	Fungal infection of the nails

which, if detached, may leave bleeding points. Plaques vary in diameter from 2 cm or less to several cm, and are sometimes pruritic.

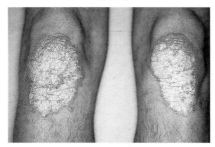

Fig. 3 **Typical scaly plaques of psoriasis on the knees.**

Guttate

Guttate psoriasis is an acute symmetrical eruption of 'drop-like' lesions usually on the trunk and limbs. The form mostly occurs in adolescents or young adults and may follow a streptococcal throat infection (Fig. 4).

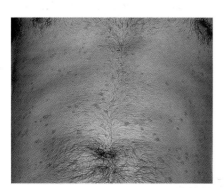

Fig. 4 **The drop-like lesions of guttate psoriasis.**

Flexural

This variant of psoriasis affects the axillae, sub-mammary areas and natal cleft (Fig. 5). Plaques are smooth and often glazed. It is mostly found in the elderly.

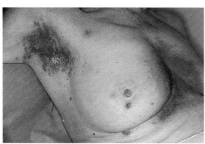

Fig. 5 **Smooth non-keratotic involvement in flexural psoriasis.**

Localized forms

Psoriasis can also present in a number of localized forms:

- *Palmoplantar pustulosis* is characterized by yellow to brown-coloured sterile pustules on the palms or soles (Fig. 6). A minority of subjects have classic plaque psoriasis elsewhere. It is most common in middle-aged females, nearly all of whom are cigarette smokers, and it follows a protracted course.
- *Acrodermatitis of Hallopeau* is an uncommon indolent form of psoriasis affecting the digits and nails (see p. 29, Fig. 3).
- *Scalp psoriasis* may be the sole manifestation of the disease (see Fig. 2, p. 29). It can be confused with dandruff but is generally better demarcated and more thickly scaled.
- *Napkin psoriasis* is a well-defined psoriasiform eruption in the nappy

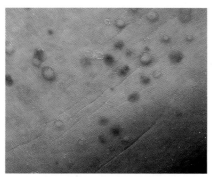

Fig. 6 **Palmoplantar pustulosis: a localized variant of psoriasis on the sole of the foot.**

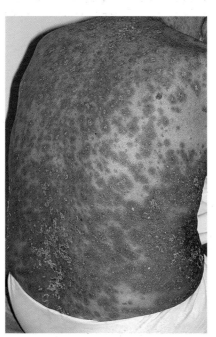

Fig. 7 **Generalized pustular psoriasis in an elderly patient.**

area of infants, some of whom later develop true psoriasis.

Generalized pustular

Generalized pustular is a rare but serious and even life-threatening form of psoriasis. Sheets of small, sterile yellowish pustules develop on an erythematous background and may rapidly spread (Fig. 7). The onset is often acute. The patient is unwell, with fever and malaise, and requires hospital admission.

Nail involvment

Psoriasis affects the matrix or nail bed in up to 50% of cases (Fig. 8). Thimble pitting is the commonest change, followed by *onycholysis* (separation of the distal edge of the nail from the nail bed). An oily or salmon pink discoloration of the nail bed is seen, often adjacent to onycholysis. Subungual hyperkeratosis, with a build-up of keratin beneath the distal nail edge, mostly affects the toe nails. Nail changes are frequently associated with psoriatic arthropathy. Treatment is often difficult.

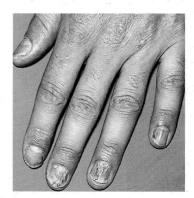

Fig. 8 **Nail involvement in psoriasis.**

Psoriasis

- Psoriasis affects 2% of the population.
- Inheritance is polygenic: 35% have a family history.
- Peak onset is in the 2nd and 3rd decades.
- Epidermal cell proliferation rate is increased, but the epidermal turnover time is reduced.
- Presentation is variable: the chronic plaque form affecting the elbows, knees and scalp is the commonest.
- Nail involvement is frequent.

PSORIASIS — Complications and Management

COMPLICATIONS

Psoriasis may be complicated by the development of arthropathy, erythroderma and the Koebner phenomenon (p. 26, Fig. 2).

Psoriatic arthropathy

Psoriatic joint disease occurs in about 5% of psoriasis patients. It shows an equal sex ratio and takes four forms:

- *Distal arthritis* is the commonest pattern. It causes swelling of the terminal interphalangeal joints of the hands and feet, sometimes with a flexion deformity. Sausage-like swelling of the digits may result.
- *Rheumatoid-like arthritis* mimics rheumatoid disease with a polyarthropathy, but is less symmetrical and the rheumatoid factor test is negative.
- *Mutilans arthritis* is often associated with severe psoriasis (Fig. 1). Erosions develop in the small bones of the hands and feet, and sometimes the spine. The bones may be dissolved giving progressive deformity.
- *Ankylosing spondylitis/sacroiliitis.* Patients with this pattern are usually positive for HLA-B27.

Erythrodermic psoriasis

Inpatient treatment is needed for this condition, often with systemic drugs. Details are given on page 40.

MANAGEMENT

The non-infectious nature of psoriasis and the likely need for long-term therapy should be explained. A sympathetic approach is helpful and patients often obtain support from the self-help group, The Psoriasis Association (see p. 120). Treatment is tailored to the patient's particular require-ments, taking into account the type and extent of the disease, and the age and social background (Table 1).

Topical therapy

It is usual to prescribe topical agents as the first line treatment.

Tar preparations

Coal-tar distillates have been used for decades to treat psoriasis. They are safe and seem to act by inhibiting DNA synthesis. The main disadvantages of tar are that it smells and is messy. Despite these, it is useful for inpatient care, especially in combination with ultraviolet B, a treatment known as the Goeckermann regimen. Refined tar is available in cream or ointment bases for out-patient use (e.g. Alphosyl, Carbo-Dome, Clinitar, Pragmatar). These preparations, which contain 1 and 10% tar, are suitable for chronic plaque psoriasis or guttate psoriasis once the acute phase is past.

Dithranol (Anthralin)

Dithranol has an anti-mitotic effect and is irritant to normal skin. It cannot be used on the face or genitalia, and it stains skin, hair, linen, clothes and bathtubs a purple-brown colour. For inpatient use, the usual base is Lassar's paste (zinc and salicylic acid paste BP). It is applied to the plaques of psoriasis initially in the 0.1% strength, increasing up to 2% if necessary. The surrounding skin is sometimes protected with a bland preparation such as white soft paraffin, and the treated area is covered with tube gauze. The combination of this with a daily tar bath and ultravio-let B is called the Ingram regimen. Psoriasis clears within 3 weeks in most patients on this treatment.

Dithranol only needs to be applied for 30 mins each day to have an effect. This 'short contact' regimen is particularly suitable for outpatient and is the treatment of choice for stable plaque psoriasis. The dithranol is best washed off in a shower as removal is more complete than in a bath and staining is less of a problem. Dithrocream is a suitable preparation and comes in concentrations from 0.1 to 2%.

Topical corticosteroids

Topical steroids have the advantage of being clean, non-irritant and easy to use. However, against this must be balanced the risk of side-effects (p. 21) and of precipitating an unstable form of psoriasis, especially on their withdrawal. Topical steroids are the treatment of choice for face, genitalia and flexures, and are useful for stubborn plaques on hands, feet and scalp. Potent steroids should not be applied to the face, although they may be used judiciously on palms and soles. Elsewhere, moderately potent steroids normally suffice. Their use must be monitored carefully. Creams are often preferred to ointments. Lotions and gels are available for the scalp.

Vitamin D analogues

Calcipotriol (Dovonex) and *tacalcitol* (Curatoderm) are topical synthetic vitamin D analogues for use in mild and moderate chronic plaque psoriasis. They inhibit cell proliferation and stimulate keratinocyte differentiation, correcting some of the epidermal cell

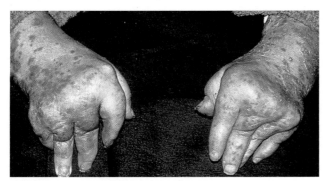

Fig. 1 **Mutilans arthropathy in severe psoriasis.**

Table 1 **A guide to psoriasis therapy**

Type of psoriasis	Treatment options
Stable plaque	Dithranol (short contact) Coal tar, vitamin D analogues UVB
Extensive plaque	PUVA (and Re-PUVA) Methotrexate, cyclosporin
Guttate	Coal tar Topical steroids (mild/moderate) UVB
Facial/flexural	Topical steroids (mild/moderate) Tacalcitol
Palmoplantar	Topical steroids (potent) Acitretin PUVA (and Re-PUVA)
Generalized pustular/ erythrodermic	Acitretin Methotrexate, cyclosporin

turnover abnormalities in psoriasis. Patient acceptability is good as the preparations do not smell or stain, are easy to apply, and do not have the risk of skin atrophy seen with topical steroids. Skin irritation may be a problem. Efficacy is commensurate with dithranol or topical steroids.

Hypercalcaemia is possible if the maximum dose is exceeded. Calcipotriol ointment or cream can be used up to 100g/week (40% of the body surface on a twice daily basis), and tacalcitol ointment up to 35g/week (20% of body surface as a once daily dose). Tacalcitol is tolerated on the face, where calcipotriol tends to irritate. Calcipotriol is available as a scalp preparation.

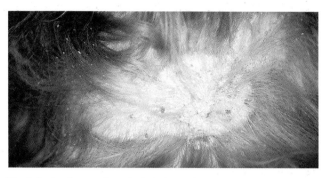

Fig. 2 **Scaly plaques of psoriasis in the scalp, with localized hair loss.**

Keratolytics and scalp preparations

Hyperkeratotic psoriasis of the palms and soles can be treated with 5% salicylic acid ointment. Scalp psoriasis (Fig. 2) responds to 3% salicylic acid in a cream base (sometimes with 3% precipitated sulphur) applied daily or every 2 or 3 days, and used in combination with a tar-containing shampoo (e.g. Alphosyl, Gelcotar, Polytar, T/Gel). Coconut oil compound (Cocois) is also helps scaly scalps.

Systemic therapy

Psoriasis that is life threatening, unresponsive to adequate topical treatment or restricting the ability to work (Fig. 3) may require systemic therapy. Benefits must be weighed against side-effects. The use of potentially toxic drugs is justified by their ability to transform a patient's life from severely restricted to nearly normal. Phototherapy and photochemotherapy are outlined on p. 100.

Methotrexate

The folate antagonist methotrexate is well established as an effective treatment for severe psoriasis and may have anti-inflammatory as well as immune modulatory effects. It is given once a week orally as a single dose (usually 7.5–15 mg), although it

can be given intramuscularly (or intravenously). Normal liver, kidney and bone marrow function must be established before starting methotrexate, and these functions must be monitored during treatment. Liver disease, alcoholism and acute infection are contra-indications to methotrexate, and drug interaction (e.g. with aspirin, non-steroidal anti-inflammatory drugs or co-trimoxazole) must be avoided. Improvement is seen within 2 to 4 weeks. Minor side-effects (e.g. nausea) are common, but liver fibrosis or cirrhosis is risk longterm. At present, this can only be detected by liver biopsy which is performed after every 1.5 g cumulative dose. Methotrexate is also a teratogen.

Retinoids

The vitamin A derivative, acitretin (Neotigason), is particularly effective in treating pustular psoriasis and in thinning hyperkeratotic plaques. Acitretin may be used with topical therapies, and UVB or PUVA ('Re–PUVA') when it allows a more rapid clearance at a lower total dose of UV. Most patients develop minor side-effects, such as dry mucous membranes (cracked lips), itching and peeling skin, but more serious complications include hyperostosis, abnor-

mal liver function, hyperlipidaemia and teratogenicity. The latter virtually precludes the use of acitretin in women of child-bearing age. Although acitretin has a half-life of 50 days, in some patients it is metabolized to etretinate, a retinoid which takes 2 years to be eliminated from the body.

Cyclosporin

Cyclosporin (Neoral), an immunosuppressant widely used to prevent rejection of organ transplants, is effective in severe psoriasis. It acts by inhibiting T-lymphocyte activation and interleukin-2 production. Dose-dependent (and reversible) nephrotoxicity is a side-effect. Blood pressure and kidney function need to be monitored during treatment. There may be a risk of skin cancers or lymphoma, and concomitant UV treatment is avoided.

Other systemic treatments

Other cytotoxic or immunosuppressive drugs may control psoriasis, but they are not as potent as methotrexate. Hydroxyurea has the advantage of not affecting the liver, but it can suppress the bone marrow. Azathioprine is both myelosuppressive and hepatotoxic.

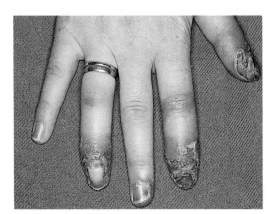

Fig. 3 **Acrodermatitis continua variant of psoriasis.** Sterile pustular changes with dactylitis are present on three fingers.

Treatment of psoriasis

Side-effects are often the limiting factor in psoriasis treatment

Topical Rx: usually the first approach

- *Coal tar:* safe but messy.
- *Dithranol:* effective but irritant.
- *Steroids:* popular but beware of side-effects.
- *Vitamin D analogues:* clean, effective, free of steroid side-effects.
- *Keratolytics:* useful for scalp involvement.

Systemic Rx: for serious or severe psoriasis

- *PUVA:* popular but long-term risk of skin cancer.
- *Retinoids:* good for pustular and as Re-PUVA; teratogenic.
- *Methotrexate:* a well-established systemic drug; hepatotoxic.
- *Cyclosporin:* effective but potentially nephrotoxic.

ECZEMA — Basic Principles/Contact Dermatitis

DEFINITION

Eczema is a non-infective inflammatory condition of the skin. The term 'eczema' literally means 'to boil over' (Greek), and this well describes the acute eruption in which blistering occurs.

Eczema represents a reaction pattern to a variety of stimuli, some of which are recognized but many of which are unknown. Eczema and dermatitis mean the same thing and may be used interchangeably. However, to patients, the term 'dermatitis' often implies an industrial causation, and its use may unnecessarily raise the question of litigation and compensation.

CLASSIFICATION

The current classification of eczema is unsatisfactory in that it is inconsistent. However, it is difficult to provide a suitable alternative since the aetiology of most eczemas is not known. Different types of eczema may be recognized either by morphology, site or cause. A division into endogenous (due to internal or constitutional factors) and exogenous (due to external contact agents) is convenient (Table 1). However, in clinical practice these distinctions are often blurred and, not infrequently, the eczema cannot be classified. A further

Table 1 **A classification of eczema**

Type	Variety
Exogenous (contact)	Allergic, irritant Photoreaction
Endogenous	Atopic Seborrhoeic Discoid (nummular) Venous (stasis, gravitational) Pompholyx
Unclassified	Asteatotic (eczema craquelé) Lichen simplex (neuro-dermatitis) Juvenile plantar dermatosis

division into acute (Fig. 1) and chronic eczema (Fig. 2) can be made in many cases according to the morphology of the eruption.

Acute eczema

In acute eczema epidermal oedema (spongiosis), with separation of keratinocytes, leads to the formation of epidermal vesicles (Fig. 3a). Dermal vessels are dilated and inflammatory cells invade the dermis and epidermis.

Chronic eczema

In chronic eczema there is thickening of the prickle cell layer (acanthosis) and stratum corneum (hyperkeratosis) with retention of nuclei by some corneocytes (parakeratosis) (Fig. 3b). The rete ridges are lengthened, dermal vessels dilated and inflamma-

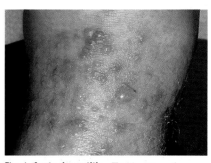

Fig. 1 **Acute dermatitis.** Erythema and oedema are seen with papules, vesicles and sometimes large blisters. Exudation and crust formation follow. The eruption is painful and pruritic. This case was due to a contact allergy to a locally applied cream.

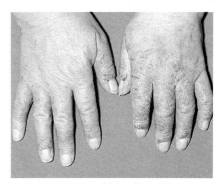

Fig. 2 **Chronic dermatitis.** Lichenification, scaling and fissuring of the hands due to repeated exposure to irritants. Allergic contact dermatitis cannot be excluded on the appearance alone.

tory mononuclear cells infiltrate the skin.

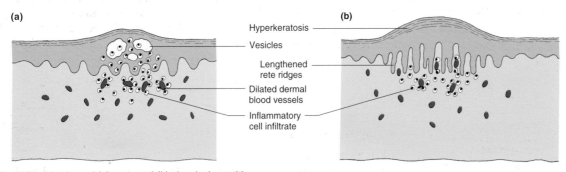

(a)   (b)

Hyperkeratosis

Vesicles

Lengthened rete ridges

Dilated dermal blood vessels

Inflammatory cell infiltrate

Fig. 3 **The histology of (a) acute and (b) chronic dermatitis.**

CONTACT DERMATITIS

DEFINITION

Dermatitis precipitated by an exogenous agent, often a chemical, is known as contact dermatitis. It is particularly common in the home, amongst women with young children, and in industry where it is a major cause of loss of time from work (see p. 116).

AETIOPATHOGENESIS

Irritants cause more cases of contact dermatitis than do allergens, although the clinical appearances are often similar. Allergic contact dermatitis is an example of type IV hypersensitivity (p. 11).

Irritants cause dermatitis in a number of different ways,

but usually by a direct noxious effect on the skin's barrier function. The most important irritants are:

- water
- abrasives
- chemicals, e.g. acids and alkalis
- solvents and detergents.

A strong irritant causing necrosis of epidermal cells will produce a reaction within hours, but in most cases the effect is more chronic. Repetitive and cumulative exposure over several months or years to water, abrasives and chemicals can induce a dermatitis, commonly on the hands. Individuals with a history of atopic eczema are more susceptible to irritants.

CLINICAL PRESENTATION

Contact dermatitis may affect any part of the body, although the hands and face are common sites. The appearance of a dermatitis at a particular site (Fig. 4) suggests contact with certain objects. For example, an eczema on the wrist of a woman with a history of reacting to cheap earrings suggests a nickel allergic response to a watch strap buckle (Fig. 5). Diagnosis is often not easy as a history of irritant or allergen exposure is not always forthcoming. Knowing the patient's occupation, hobbies, past history and use of cosmetics or medicaments helps in listing possible causes.

Nickel sensitivity is the commonest contact allergy, affecting 10% of women and 1% of men. Usually it only causes an inconvenient eczema at jewellery or metal contact sites, but an industrial dermatitis can result, e.g. in nickel platers.

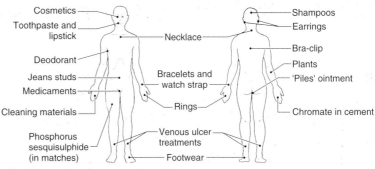
Fig. 4 **Distribution clues for contact dermatitis.**

Environmental sources of common allergens are shown in Table 2. Medicaments (p. 17) and cosmetics (p. 102) can also induce allergic or irritant reactions. Allergic contact dermatitis occasionally becomes generalized by secondary 'autosensitization' spread. Activation by ultraviolet radiation of a topically or systemically administered agent produces a photocontact reaction (p. 43).

DIFFERENTIAL DIAGNOSIS

Contact dermatitis of the hands needs to be differentiated from endogenous eczema, psoriasis and fungal infection. Acute contact dermatitis of the face may resemble angioedema or erysipelas.

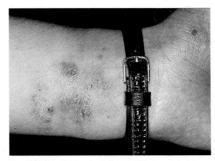
Fig. 5 **Allergic contact dermatitis to nickel in a watch strap buckle.**

MANAGEMENT

The management of contact dermatitis is not always easy because of the many and often overlapping factors which can be involved in any one case. The *identification* of any offending allergen or irritant is the overriding objective. *Patch testing* (p. 118) helps identify any allergens involved and is particularly useful in dermatitis of the face, hands and feet. The exclusion of an offending allergen from the environment is desirable, and if this can be achieved, the dermatitis may clear.

However, it is difficult to fully eliminate all contact with ubiquitous allergens such as nickel or colophony. Similarly irritants are often impossible to exclude. Some contact with irritants may be inevitable due to the nature of certain jobs, but work practices can be improved. Unnecessary contact with irritants should be limited, protective clothing worn (notably PVC gloves) and adequate washing and drying facilities provided. *Barrier creams* are seldom the answer, although they do encourage personal skin care. *Topical steroids* (moderately potent or potent) help in contact dermatitis but are secondary to avoidance measures.

Table 2 **The sources of common allergens**

Allergen	Source
Chromate	Cement, tanned leather, primer paint, anticorrosives
Cobalt	Pigment, paint, ink, metal alloys
Colophony	Glue, plasticizer, adhesive tape, varnish, polish
Epoxy resins	Adhesive, plastics, mouldings
Fragrance	Cosmetics, creams, soaps, detergents
Nickel	Jewellery, zips, fasteners, scissors, instruments
Paraphenylenediamine	Dye (clothing, hair), shoes, colour developer
Plants	*Primula obconica*, chrysanthemums, garlic, poison ivy/oak (USA)
Preservatives	Cosmetics, creams and oils
Rubber chemicals	Tyres, boots, shoes, belts, condoms, gloves

Contact Dermatitis

- *Irritants* cause more contact dermatitis than do allergens.
- *Irritant contact dermatitis*, in many cases, cannot be distinguished from allergic on morphological grounds alone.
- *Atopics* are more susceptible to the effects of irritants.
- *Patch testing* is helpful to confirm allergic contact dermatitis, particularly of the face, hands and feet.
- *Common allergens*: nickel, chromates, cobalt, colophony, preservatives, fragrance, and paraphenylenediamine.
- *Common irritants*: water, abrasives, chemicals (especially alkalis), solvents, oils, and detergents.
- *Elimination and avoidance* of allergens and irritants are useful although prevention is the ideal.

ECZEMA — Atopic Eczema

DEFINITION

Atopic eczema is a chronic pruritic inflammation of the epidermis and dermis, often associated with a personal or family history of asthma, allergic rhinitis, conjunctivitis or atopic eczema. Uncontrollable scratching is prominent and the course is remitting.

AETIOPATHOGENESIS

'Atopy' defines an inherited tendency (p. 12), present in 15–25% of the population, to develop one or more of the aforementioned disorders and to produce high levels of circulating IgE antibodies, commonly to inhalant allergens (e.g. housedust mite). Excessive IgE production is not the primary abnormality but is the result of a more fundamental imbalance of immune function; this includes defective T cell function as shown by a decreased capacity to produce certain cytokines. The basic cause of the atopic eczema lesion is still uncertain, although recent evidence suggests that the housedust mite antigen is important in some cases.

INCIDENCE

About 12–15% of infants are affected. It usually starts within the first 6 months of life, and by 1 year, 60% of those likely to develop it will have done so. Two-thirds have a family history of atopy. Remission occurs by the age of 15 years in 75%, although some relapse later.

CLINICAL PRESENTATION

The appearance of atopic eczema differs depending on the age of the patient.

Infancy

Babies develop an itchy vesicular exudative eczema on the face (Fig. 1) and hands, often with secondary infection. Less than half continue to have eczema beyond 18 months.

Childhood

After 18 months, the pattern often changes to the familiar involvement of the antecubital and popliteal fossae, neck, wrists and ankles (Figs 2 and 3). The face often shows erythema and infraorbital folds. Lichenification,

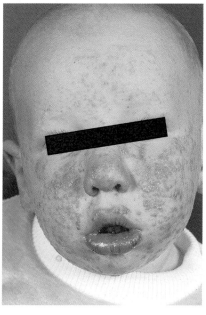

Fig. 1 **Atopic eczema in an infant.** Secondary bacterial infection was present.

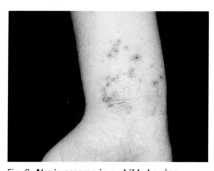

Fig. 2 **Atopic eczema in a child showing excoriations and lichenification at the wrist.**

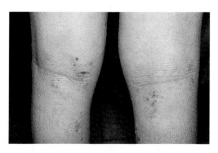

Fig. 3 **Atopic eczema involving the popliteal fossa in a child.**

excoriations and dry skin (Fig. 4) are common, and palmar markings may be increased. Post-inflammatory hyperpigmentation occurs in those with a pigmented skin. Scratching or rubbing cause most of the clinical signs and are particularly a problem at night when they can interfere with sleep. Hyperactivity is sometimes seen, and the child may use his or her eczema to manipulate the family.

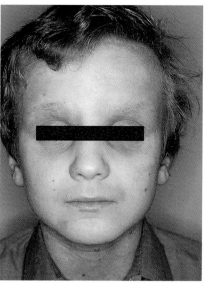

Fig. 4 **A 'dry' pruritic type of atopic eczema.** Note the loss of eyebrows due to constant rubbing.

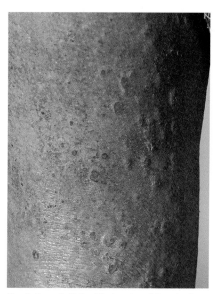

Fig. 5 **Grossly lichenified and nodular atopic eczema in an adult.**

Schoolchildren with eczema may be teased or rejected by their classmates.

Adults

The commonest manifestation in adult life is hand dermatitis, exacerbated by irritants, in someone with a past history of atopic eczema. However, a small number of adults have a chronic severe form of generalized and lichenified atopic eczema (Fig. 5) which may interfere with their employment and social activities. Stressful situations, such as examinations or marital problems, often coincide with exacerbations.

DIFFERENTIAL DIAGNOSIS

Infantile flexural eczema may sometimes develop into the atopic variety, and occasionally the distinction from scabies is necessary. Rarely, infants with immune deficiency syndromes (e.g. Wiskott-Aldrich), or with histiocytosis X, have an eczematous eruption.

INVESTIGATIONS

Prick tests to inhalant and (sometimes) food allergens are frequently positive, indicating type I hypersensitivity (p. 118). Total serum IgE levels are raised in 80% of patients and the radioallergoabsorbance test (RAST) may be positive for specific allergens. These tests are rarely needed to make the diagnosis. Swabs for bacterial and viral culture may be helpful during an exacerbation.

COMPLICATIONS

Atopic eczema is subject to several complications — some common and some rare:

- *Bacterial infection.* Secondary infection (usually with *Staphylococcus aureus*) commonly causes an exacerbation.
- *Viral infection.* Patients have an increased susceptibility to infection with viral warts and molluscum contagiosum.
- *Eczema herpeticum.* There is a propensity to develop widespread lesions with herpes simplex (Fig.6) and vaccinia.
- *Cataracts.* A specific form of cataract infrequently develops in young adults with severe atopic eczema.
- *Growth retardation.* Children with severe atopic eczema may have short stature. Usually the cause is unknown.
- *Ichthyosis vulgaris.* More common in patients with atopic eczema.

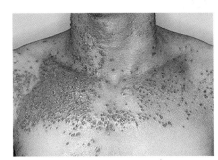

Fig. 6 **Eczema herpeticum.** Herpes simplex infection complicating atopic eczema.

MANAGEMENT

General measures in the management of atopic eczema include explaining the disorder and its treatment to the patient and the parents, stressing the normally good prognosis. A child should wear loose cotton clothing and avoid wool (which irritates) and excessive heat. Nails should be kept short. Cats and dogs cause exacerbations in some patients and are best kept away. The exclusion of housedust mite from the home environment is difficult. Careers advice is also important. Wetwork jobs (e.g. nursing, hairdressing, cleaning) and industrial work with exposure to irritant oils should be avoided. Some sufferers obtain support from groups such as the National Eczema Society (p. 120). Specialist nurses are skilful in managing eczema patients.

Specific treatments for atopic eczema are summarized in Table 1.

Table 1 **Treatment of atopic eczema**

Treatment	Indication
Emollients	Most eczema; ichthyosis
Topical steroids	Most types of eczema
Tar bandage	Lichenified/excoriated eczema
Oral antihistamine	Pruritus
Oral antibiotic	Bacterial superinfection
Exclusion diet	Food allergy/resistant eczema
PUVA	Very resistant eczema
Cyclosporin	Resistant severe eczema

Topical therapy

Emollients
Emollients such as aqueous cream and emulsifying ointment should be used regularly on the skin and as soap substitutes. They moisturize the dry skin, diminishing the desire to scratch and reducing the need for topical steroids. Bath oil emollients may also help.

Topical steroids
The rule is to prescribe the least potent strength steroid that is effective. In children, 1% hydrocortisone ointment applied twice a day is usually adequate (ointments are generally preferred to creams for eczema). Sometimes it is necessary to use a moderately potent steroid for a short time in children with resistant eczema, and for rather more prolonged periods in adults with established and severe eczema.

Topical antibiotics or antiseptics
Topical antibiotics or antiseptics may be used for infected eczema, either in combination with a steroid (e.g. Fucibet cream) or separately (e.g. Bactroban or Fucidin ointment).

Coal tar or ichthammol paste
Coal tar or ichthammol paste is useful for lichenified or excoriated eczema and may be prescribed as an occlusive medicated bandage (e.g. Coltapaste or Ichthopaste) which is normally left on overnight.

Wet dressings
Wet wraps are often required for a short time on an exudative eczema.

Systemic therapy
A sedative antihistamine, such as promethazine or trimeprazine, given at night, helps to reduce the desire to scratch in both children and adults. Infected exacerbations frequently require the intermittent use of an antibiotic by mouth, and flucloxacillin is often selected. Eczema herpeticum is usually an indication for admission to hospital (with appropriate isolation of the patient); treatment is with aciclovir (Zovirax). Patients with the most severe and resistant forms of atopic eczema may be treated with PUVA (p. 101), or cyclosporin (p. 107), given as an 8 week course.

Dietary manipulation
Some children with atopic eczema give a history that suggests food allergy (e.g. urticaria of the mouth on contact with the food, or gastrointestinal symptoms) and it is clear that the offending food should be avoided. Otherwise, dietary treatment is reserved for a minority who have not improved with standard therapy. Diets free from cows' milk or eggs may be tried but must be supervised by a dietician to ensure exclusion and to prevent nutritional deficiencies.

Atopic eczema
- Affects 12–15% of infants (usual onset less than 1 year old).
- Aetiology is not well understood but immune function is disturbed.
- Classically affects face, and knee and elbow flexures.
- Itch-scratch cycle induces lichenification.
- Exacerbations are often due to infection, particularly staphylococcal.
- Treatment involves emollients, topical steroids, tar bandages, systemic antihistamines and antibiotics.

ECZEMA — Other forms

The other main types of eczema are seborrhoeic, discoid, venous, asteatotic and hand dermatitis.

SEBORRHOEIC DERMATITIS

Seborrhoeic dermatitis is a chronic, scaly inflammatory eruption usually affecting the scalp and face.

Aetiopathogenesis

Sebum production is normal, but the eruption often occurs in the sebaceous gland areas of the scalp, face and chest. Endogenous and genetic factors, and an overgrowth of the commensal yeast *Pityrosporum ovale*, seem to be involved. The condition is severe in some patients with AIDS.

Clinical presentation

There are four common patterns:

- *Scalp and facial involvement:* excessive dandruff, with an itchy scaly erythematous eruption affecting the sides of the nose, scalp margin, eyebrows and ears (Fig.1). Blepharitis may occur. Most common in young adult males.
- *Petaloid:* a dry scaly eczema over the presternal area.
- *Pityrosporum folliculitis:* an erythematous follicular eruption with papules or pustules over the back (Fig. 2).
- *Flexural:* involvement of the axillae, groins and sub-mammary

areas by a moist intertrigo, often secondarily colonized by *Candida albicans*. Seen in the elderly (do not confuse with the similarly named infantile eruption. p. 108).

Management

The scalp lesions require the use of a medicated shampoo (e.g. containing coal tar, selenium sulphide or ketoconazole), either alone or following the application of 2% sulphur and 2% salicylic acid cream left on for several hours. Facial, truncal and flexural involvement responds to an imidazole or antimicrobial, often combined with 1% hydrocortisone, in a cream or ointment base (e.g. Daktacort and Vioform-Hydrocortisone). Lithium succinate (Efalith) cream is also effective. Recurrence is common and repeated treatment often necessary.

DISCOID (NUMMULAR) ECZEMA

Discoid eczema is an eczema of

Table 1 **Differential diagnosis of seborrhoeic dermatitis**

Site of seborrhoeic dermatitis	Differential diagnosis
Face	Psoriasis, contact dermatitis, rosacea
Scalp	Psoriasis, fungal infection
Trunk	Psoriasis, pityriasis versicolor, Fungal infection

unknown aetiology characterized by coin-shaped lesions on the limbs; it typically affects middle-aged or elderly men (Fig. 3). Younger subjects may have atopic eczema.

Clinical presentation

The coin-shaped eczema lesions are often symmetrical and can be intensely itchy. The eczema may be vesicular or chronic and lichenified. It may clear after a few weeks but tends to recur. Secondary bacterial infection is common.

Management

The condition can often be confused with tinea corporis and contact dermatitis.

A moderately potent or potent topical steroid, often combined with an antimicrobial or antibiotic, is helpful.

VENOUS (STASIS) ECZEMA

Venous eczema affects the lower legs (Fig. 4) and is associated with underlying venous disease (p. 68). Incompetence of the deep perforating veins increases the hydrostatic pressure in the dermal capillaries. Peri-capillary fibrin deposition leads to the clinical changes.

Clinical presentation

Most patients are middle-aged or elderly women. Leashes of venules and haemosiderin pigmentation around the ankles are early signs.

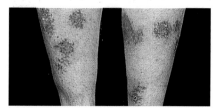

Fig. 3 **Discoid eczema of the lower leg.**

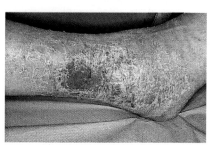

Fig. 4 **Venous eczema.**

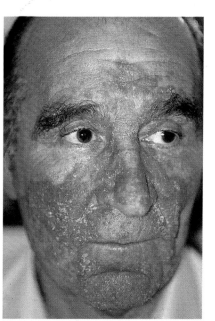

Fig. 1 **Seborrhoeic dermatitis affecting the face.**

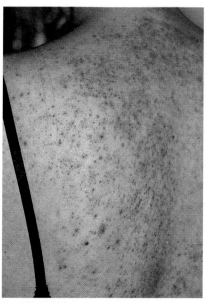

Fig. 2 **Seborrhoeic dermatitis of the pityrosporum folliculitis type affecting the back.**

Eczema develops, sometimes with fibrosis of the dermis and subcutaneous tissue (lipodermatosclerosis), and ulceration. Allergy to an applied medicament can complicate the picture.

Management

An emollient, alone or with a mild or moderately potent steroid ointment, is needed. Tar-impregnated bandages (e.g. Ichthopaste or Coltapaste), applied once or twice a week, are useful especially when ulceration coexists. Venous disease or ulceration is treated on its own merit (p. 69).

HAND DERMATITIS

Hand dermatitis is a common, often recurrent condition which varies from being acute and vesicular to chronic, hyperkeratotic and fissured. The condition results from a variety of causes, and often several factors are involved. In children, hand dermatitis is mostly due to atopic eczema. An atopic predisposition often underlies adult hand dermatitis, especially if due to repeated exposure to irritants.

Allergic causes need excluding, and most adults with hand dermatitis require patch testing. Fungal infection is ruled out by microscopy and culture, especially in unilateral hand dermatitis, and the feet are examined since tinea pedis can provoke a hand dermatitis as an 'id' phenomenon (p. 54). A core of patients is left who have an endogenous recurrent hand dermatitis often characterized by sago-like vesicles on the sides of the fingers, on the palms and sometimes the soles.

Clinical presentation

Hand dermatitis often presents as a chronic eczema, but may appear as a vesicular eruption known as *pompholyx*. Vesicles may be seen with atopic eczema or contact dermatitis,

Table 2 **Hints on hand care for hand dermatitis patients**

Hand washing
Use warm water and unscented soap, and avoid paper towels; use a dry cotton towel

Protection
Avoid wetwork if possible, or otherwise wear cotton gloves under PVC gloves; wear gloves in cold weather and for dusty work

Medicaments
Use emollients regularly throughout the day; apply steroid ointments twice a day

Avoid handling
Shampoos, hair preparations, detergents, solvents, polishes, certain vegetables (e.g. tomatoes, potatoes), peeling fruits (e.g. oranges) and cutting meats

but in pompholyx there is usually no associated disorder. The onset is in young adults, particularly in warm weather, and it is often recurrent. Involvement can be confined to a few microvesicles on the fingers, or can be extensive with bullae affecting the whole hand (Fig. 5). Some patients are nickel-sensitive.

Management

Acute pompholyx requires drainage of large blisters and the application (once or twice a day) of wet dressings (e.g. immersed in 0.01% aqueous potassium permanganate, 0.5% aqueous silver nitrate or Burow's solution of 0.65% aqueous aluminium acetate). Oral antibiotics are given if bacterial infection is present. Some dermatologists prescribe systemic steroids, but these are usually not necessary. Once the acute stage settles, potent or highly potent steroid lotions or creams are used with cotton gloves. For chronic or subacute cases, a steroid ointment and emollients are helpful. Advice for patients with hand dermatitis is given in Table 2.

ASTEATOTIC ECZEMA (ECZEMA CRAQUELÉ)

Asteatotic eczema is a dry eczema with fissuring and cracking of the skin, often affecting limbs in the elderly (Fig. 6).

Overwashing of patients in institutions, a dry winter climate, hypothyroidism and use of diuretics, can contribute to eczema in elderly

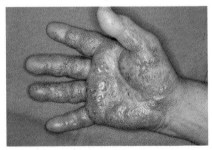

Fig. 5 **Acute pompholyx involving the entire palmar surface of the hand in a nickel-sensitive woman.**

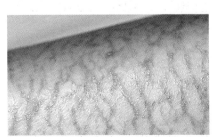

Fig. 6 **Asteatotic eczema.**

atrophic skin. The skin of the limbs and trunk is erythematous, dry and itchy and shows a fine crazy-paving pattern of fissuring. Emollients applied to the skin and used in the bath often suffice to clear up the condition, but sometimes a mild steroid is necessary.

OTHER ECZEMAS

Other types of eczema are occasionally encountered. They include: lichen simplex chronicus, lichen striatus, juvenile plantar dermatosis (p. 108) and napkin (diaper) eruption (p. 108).

Lichen simplex chronicus (neurodermatitis)

Neurodermatitis is an area of lichenified eczema due to repeated rubbing or scratching, as a habit or due to 'stress'. It usually occurs as a single plaque on the lower leg, back of the neck or in the perineum (*pruritus vulvae/ani*: p. 113). The skin markings are exaggerated and pigmentation may occur. Asians and Chinese are particularly susceptible. Sometimes a nodular lichenification known as *prurigo nodularis* develops on the shins and forearms. Topical steroids, weak tar paste and tar-impregnated bandages are the mainstay of treatment.

Lichen striatus

Lichen striatus is a rare self-limiting linear eczema affecting a limb and occurring in adolescents (p. 19).

Eczema

- *Seborrhoeic dermatitis* commonly affects the scalp and face; responds to combined antimicrobial/hydrocortisone creams.
- *Discoid eczema* often presents as coin-shaped lesions on limbs of middle-aged or elderly; improves with moderate potency topical steroids.
- *Venous eczema* is associated with venous disease; responds to emollients and low or moderate potency topical steroids.
- *Hand dermatitis*: multiple and mixed aetiology; determine causes by exclusion.
- *Asteatotic eczema*: the eczema craquelé of elderly skin. Treat with emollients or low potency topical steroids.

LICHENOID ERUPTIONS

Lichen planus and other disorders with a lichenoid appearance are presented here.

LICHEN PLANUS

Lichen planus is a relatively common pruritic papular dermatosis involving the flexor surfaces, mucous membranes and genitalia.

The cause is unknown, but an immune pathogenesis is suggested by the finding of IgM at the dermo-epidermal junction and an association with some autoimmune diseases.

Pathology

In lichen planus, the granular layer is thickened, basal cells show liquefaction degeneration and lymphocytes infiltrate the upper dermis in a band-like fashion (Fig. 1).

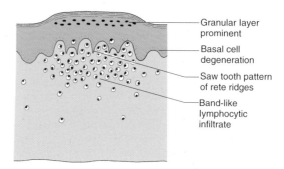

Granular layer prominent
Basal cell degeneration
Saw tooth pattern of rete ridges
Band-like lymphocytic infiltrate

Fig. 1 **Histopathology of lichen planus.**

Clinical presentation

Two-thirds of cases occur in the 30–60 year old age group. It is uncommon at the extremes of age, and the sex incidence is equal. Lichen planus tends to start on the limbs. It may spread rapidly to become generalized within 4 weeks, but the commoner localized forms progress more slowly. Typical lesions are very itchy flat-topped polygonal papules, a few mm in diameter, which may show a surface network of delicate white lines (Wickham's striae). Initially, the papules are red, but they become violaceous (Fig. 2).

The eruption is symmetrical and affects:

- forearms and wrists
- lower legs and thighs
- genitalia
- palms and soles.

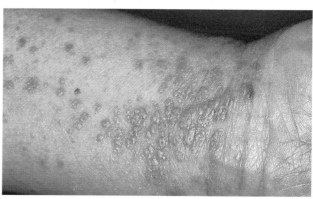

Fig. 2 **Typical violaceous papules of lichen planus at the wrist.**

Mucous membrane involvement, especially of the buccal mucosa, occurs in two-thirds of cases (Fig. 3). Lichen planus also shows the Koebner phenomenon (p. 19). Follicular and other variants are found (see below). In most cases, papules flatten after a few months to leave pigmentation, but some become hypertrophic. Half of all patients are clear within 9 months, but 15% have continuing symptoms even after 18 months. Up to 20% have a further attack. Lichen planus may be confused with other conditions as shown in Table 1.

Variants of lichen planus

A number of variants of lichen planus exist:

- *Annular:* found in 10% of cases, commonly on the glans penis.
- *Atrophic:* rare, may be seen with hypertrophic lesions.
- *Bullous:* blisters appear infrequently in lichen planus.
- *Follicular:* may occur with typical lichen planus; can affect scalp alone (scarring alopecia p. 63).
- *Hypertrophic:* verrucous plaques

affect the lower legs or arms (Fig. 4); may persist for years.

- *Mucous membrane:* any mucosal surface may be affected, with or without lesions elsewhere (Fig. 3).

Complications

Lichen planus may be complicated by:

- *Nail involvement:* found in 10% of patients. Longitudinal grooving and pitting are reversible, but dystrophic/atrophic lesions can produce scarring or permanent nail loss.

Table 1 **Differential diagnosis: lichen planus**

Type of lichen planus	Differential diagnosis
Generalized	Lichenoid drug eruption Guttate psoriasis Atypical pityriasis rosea
Genital	Psoriasis, scabies Lichen sclerosus
Hypertrophic	Lichen simplex

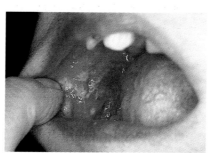

Fig. 3 **White lace-like Wickham's striae on the buccal mucosa.**

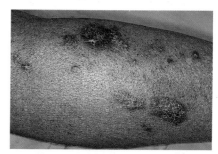

Fig. 4 **Hypertrophic lichen planus showing hyperpigmentation.**

- *Scalp lesions:* may be follicular, but pseudopelade-like permanent scarring alopecia is more common (p. 63).
- Malignant change: very infrequent.

Management

Lichen planus disease is self-limiting in most patients. Moderate to high potency topical steroids usually produce symptomatic improvement. Oral lesions are helped by a steroid-containing paste (e.g. Adcortyl in Orabase). Hypertrophic lichen planus may require highly potent topical steroids, sometimes under occlusion, or intralesional steroid injection. Extensive involvement, ulcerative mucous membrane lesions or a potentially scarring nail dystrophy warrant a trial of systemic prednisolone (in a dose of 10–40mg/d) for 1 to 3 months. Long-term systemic steroids are not justified. PUVA may help resistant cases.

LICHEN SCLEROSUS

Lichen sclerosus is an uncommon disorder typified by white lichenoid atrophic lesions on the genitalia. Although associated with autoimmune disease, the cause is unknown.

Pathology

The epidermis may be thickened, thinned or hyperkeratotic. The upper dermis is oedematous, hyalinized and acellular. Lymphocytes infiltrate the lower dermis.

Clinical presentation

Lichen sclerosus occurs ten times more frequently in women. It is commonest in middle-age, although, it may develop in childhood (with a better prognosis). Genital lesions are almost invariable, but involvement of the trunk or arms is seen. Individual lesions are a few mm in diameter, porcelain white and slightly atrophic and may aggregate into wrinkled plaques (Fig. 5). Hyperkeratosis, telangiectasia, purpura and even blistering occur. Vulval and perianal

lesions cause itching and soreness. Involvement in the male results in urethral stricture and phimosis (balanitis xerotica obliterans). Occasionally, lesions are found in the mouth. Lichen sclerosus is chronic and usually permanent. Spontaneous resolution is most likely at puberty in childhood cases.

Differential diagnosis

Female genital involvement may resemble lichen simplex chronicus (p. 35), Bowen's disease (p. 98), and extra-mammary Paget's disease. Male genital lesions mimic lichen planus, psoriasis and some rare inflammatory and premalignant forms of balanitis (p. 113).

Complications

Dysuria and dyspareunia are a problem in females, and males may experience recurrent balanitis and ulceration of the glans. Squamous cell carcinoma develops infrequently in the longstanding lesions of both sexes.

Management

Non-genital lesions require no treatment. In female genital involvement, a mild- to moderate-potency steroid cream (with or without an antiseptic/antibiotic) will reduce the itch. Vulvectomy is contraindicated in uncomplicated cases.

Treatment is similar for the male genital lesions, although circumcision is performed if phimosis develops. Both sexes need long-term follow-up and biopsy of any suspicious areas.

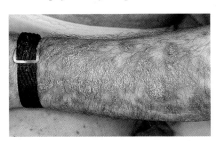

Fig. 6 **A lichenoid drug eruption, here due to quinine.**

Table 2 **Drugs causing a lichen planus-like eruption**

Type of agent	Drug
Antiarthritic	Gold, penicillamine
Antibiotic	Streptomycin, tetracycline
Antimalarial	Chloroquine, mepacrine, quinine
Antituberculous	PAS, isoniazid, ethambutol
Diuretic	Thiazides, frusemide
ACE inhibitor	Captopril
Antidiabetic	Tolbutamide, chlorpropamide
Antipsychotic	Phenothiazines

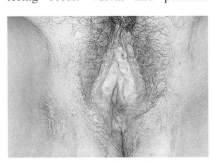

Fig. 5 **Lichen sclerosus.**

LICHEN NITIDUS

Lichen nitidus is an uncommon eruption of minute monomorphic flesh-coloured papules. The aetiology is unknown. Histology reveals a lymphohistiocytic infiltrate which expands a single dermal papilla.

Clinical presentation and management

The eruption is asymptomatic, often noticed by chance, and usually occurs in children or young adults. Uniform pinhead-sized papules, which may be grouped, are seen on the forearms, penis, abdomen and buttocks. The main differential diagnosis is lichen planus (which may coexist with it) and keratosis pilaris (p. 86).

Treatment is usually unnecessary. Lichen nitidus may resolve in weeks or persist indefinitely.

LICHEN PLANUS-LIKE DRUG ERUPTIONS

An eruption resembling lichen planus can follow the ingestion of several drugs.

Clinical presentation

A lichen planus-like rash has been recognized with gold and mepacrine therapy for many years. The eruption, which can be severe, is often more hypertrophic and hyperpigmented than true lichen planus (Fig. 6) and, on histology, shows a greater number of eosinophils. Resolution after withdrawal of the drug is often slow. Table 2 lists some of the drugs responsible.

Lichenoid eruptions

- *Lichen planus* is a relatively common pruritic papular eruption which resolves in most cases within 18 months.
- *Lichen planus-like drug eruption* resembles lichen planus but is more persistent; it is seen, for example, with gold, chloroquine and chlorothiazide.
- *Lichen nitidus* is a rare, asymptomatic eruption of fine monomorphic papules on the abdomen, arms and penis.
- *Lichen sclerosus* is mostly found in women, and frequently affects the genitalia. Long-term follow-up is necessary due to the risk of malignant change.

PAPULOSQUAMOUS ERUPTIONS

Papulosquamous eruptions are raised, scaly and marginated, and include psoriasis, lichen planus and other conditions listed in Table 1. Eczema is not included as it does not usually have a sharp edge. These eruptions are not related aetiologically. Several are characterized by fine scaling and have the prefix 'pityriasis' which means 'bran-like scale'.

Table 1 **Papulosquamous eruptions**

Chronic superficial dermatitis	Pityriasis rubra pilaris (p. 40)
Drug eruption (p. 82)	Pityriasis versicolor
Lichen planus (p. 36)	Psoriasis (p. 26)
Pityriasis alba	Reiter's disease
Pityriasis lichenoides	Secondary syphilis
Pityriasis rosea	Tinea infection (p. 54)

PITYRIASIS ROSEA

Pityriasis rosea is an acute, self-limiting disorder of unknown aetiology characterized by scaly oval papules and plaques which mainly occur on the trunk.

Clinical presentation
The generalized eruption is preceded in most patients by the appearance of a single lesion, 2–5 cm in diameter, known as a 'herald patch' (Fig. 1). Some days later, many smaller plaques appear mainly on the trunk but also on the upper arms and thighs. Individual plaques are oval, pink and have a delicate peripheral 'collarette' of scale. They are distributed parallel to the lines of the ribs, radiating away from the spine. Itching is mild or moderate. The eruption fades spontaneously in 4–8 weeks. It tends to affect teenagers and young adults. The cause is unknown, but epidemiological evidence of 'clustering' suggests an infective aetiology.

Differential diagnosis and management
Guttate psoriasis, pityriasis versicolor and secondary syphilis may cause confusion. A serological test for syphilis is needed in doubtful cases. The condition is self-limiting and treatment does not hasten clearance, although a moderate potency topical steroid can help relieve pruritus.

PITYRIASIS (TINEA) VERSICOLOR

Pityriasis versicolor is a chronic, often asymptomatic, fungal infection characterized by pigmentary changes and involving the trunk.

Clinical presentation
The condition is caused by overgrowth of the mycelial form of the commensal yeast *Pityrosporum orbiculare* and is particularly common in humid or tropical conditions. In the UK it mainly affects young adults, appearing on the trunk and proximal parts of the limbs (Fig. 2). In untanned, white caucasians, brown or pinkish oval or round superficially scaly patches are seen, but in tanned or racially pigmented skin, hypopigmentation is found due to the release by the organism of carboxylic acids which inhibit melanogenesis.

Differential diagnosis
Differentiation from vitiligo is important: usually pityriasis versicolor has a fine scale, and scrapings readily show the 'grapes and bananas' appearance of the spores and short hyphae on microscopy. Pityriasis rosea and tinea corporis may occasionally appear similar.

Management
Treatment involves either the topical application of one of the imidazole antifungals (e.g. Canesten or Daktarin cream) or the use of 2.5% selenium sulphide (Selsun) shampoo, applied to all affected areas at night and washed off the following morning (repeated twice at weekly intervals). Itraconazole, 200 mg daily for 7 days, is effective for resistant cases. Recurrences are common.

REITER'S DISEASE

Reiter's disease is a syndrome of polyarthropathy, urethritis, iritis and a psoriasiform eruption.

Clinical presentation and management
Reiter's disease almost invariably affects males who have the HLA-B27 genotype and commonly follows a genito-urinary or bowel infection. The joint and eye changes are often severe. Skin involvement includes a balanitis (p. 113) and red, scaled, pustular, psoriasiform plaques on the feet (keratoderma blenorrhagicum).

Severe skin changes are unresponsive to topical therapy and methotrexate or retinoids are often needed.

CHRONIC SUPERFICIAL DERMATITIS

Previously known as parapsoriasis, this is an uncommon chronic dermatitis of scaly pink-coloured oval or round-shaped plaques which may be premalignant.

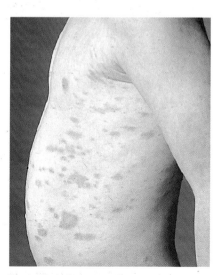

Fig. 1 **Pityriasis rosea.** Figure shows a herald patch at the lower abdomen and associated oval scaly plaques.

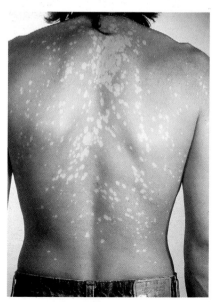

Fig. 2 **Pityriasis versicolor on the trunk revealed by tanning in the sun.**

Clinical presentation

In chronic superficial dermatitis, scaly patches develop, usually on the abdomen, buttocks or thighs. The onset is in mid- to late-adult life and the plaques are indolent. It is difficult to predict which cases will progress to mycosis fungoides (p. 98), especially since the evolution may take place over many years, but the 'benign' lesions tend to be small and finger-like in shape (Fig. 3), whereas the 'premalignant' plaques are larger, asymmetrical, atrophic and may show associated poikiloderma (reticulate pigmentation, telangiectasia and atrophy). Biopsy is necessary to look for the changes of mycosis fungoides, and further biopsy of any changed area is required.

Differential diagnosis and management

Psoriasis, discoid eczema and tinea corporis may need to be considered in diagnosis, but the plaques of chronic superficial dermatitis are distinguished by being fixed.

The first-line treatment with moderately potent topical steroids is sometimes helpful. UVB or PUVA will often be needed for a premalignant eruption. Long-term follow-up is recommended.

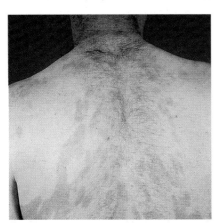

Fig. 3 **Plaques of chronic superficial dermatitis on the back of a middle-aged male.**

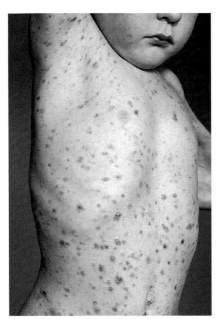

Fig. 4 **Pityriasis lichenoides (acute type) in a child.**

OTHER PITYRIASES

Other varieties of pityriasis include:

- *Pityriasis lichenoides*: a rare chronic eruption in which small papules topped by a fine single scale appear on the limbs and trunk. It is seen in adolescents and young adults and may occur in an acute form (Fig. 4) which heals with scarring.
- *Pityriasis rubra pilaris*: a rare, scaly follicular eruption which may progress to erythroderma (see p. 40).
- *Pityriasis alba*: occurs in children or young adults and is characterized by finely scaled white patches on the face or arms. It is often seen in atopics.

SECONDARY SYPHILIS

Definition

Secondary syphilis is an inflammatory response in the skin and mucous membranes to the disseminated *Treponema pallidum* spirochaete.

Clinical presentation

The secondary phase of syphilis (p. 112) starts 4–12 weeks after the appearance of the primary chancre and consists of an eruption, lymphadenopathy and variable malaise. Pink or copper-coloured macules, which later develop into papules, appear in a symmetrical distribution on the trunk and limbs and are non-itchy (Fig. 5). Annular patterns are not uncommon, and involvement of the palms and soles is distinctive. Other signs are moist warty lesions (condyloma lata) in the anogenital area, buccal erosions that may be arcuate (snail-track ulcers) and a diffuse patchy alopecia. Mucosal lesions are infectious. Without treatment, the lesions of secondary syphilis resolve spontaneously in 1–3 months.

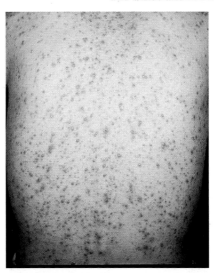

Fig. 5 **The copper, pink-coloured macules and papules of secondary syphilis on the trunk.**

Differential diagnosis and management

Pityriasis rosea, psoriasis, drug eruption, infectious mononucleosis, rubella and measles may need to be considered. Treponemal serology is positive in all patients with secondary syphilis. Treatment is with intramuscular procaine penicillin (p. 112).

Other papulosquamous eruptions

- *Pityriasis rosea* is a fairly common self-limiting eruption of young adults; scaly oval plaques follow herald patch.
- *Pityriasis versicolor* is a common truncal eruption of young adults and is due to a commensal yeast. It is often revealed in the summer as pale areas adjacent to tanned skin.
- *Reiter's syndrome* typically affects young males and follows a genitourinary or bowel infection. Keratotic skin lesions are seen with eye and joint changes.
- *Chronic superficial dermatitis* is uncommon, with middle-aged onset. Indolent plaques on trunk / limbs may progress to mycosis fungoides.
- *Pityriasis lichenoides* is a rare chronic eruption of scaly-topped papules on trunk and limbs. An acute form may scar.
- *Secondary syphilis* is a symmetrical, non-itchy truncal eruption with mucosal and palmar or plantar lesions due to infection with *T. pallidum*.

ERYTHRODERMA

DEFINITION

Erythroderma or generalized exfoliative dermatitis defines any inflammatory dermatosis which involves all or nearly all of the skin surface (sometimes stated as more than 90%). It is a secondary process and represents the generalized spread of a dermatosis or systemic disease throughout the skin.

PATHOLOGY

The duration and severity of the inflammatory process play more of a part in deciding the histology than does the underlying cause. In the acute eruption, oedema of the epidermis and dermis is prominent and there is an inflammatory infiltrate. More chronic lesions show lengthened rete ridges and thickening of the epidermis. Abnormal lymphocytes eventually may be apparent in those cases due to lymphoma, and specific changes identified on biopsy of a typical lesion when either psoriasis, ichthyosiform erythroderma or pityriasis rubra pilaris is the cause.

CLINICAL PRESENTATION

Erythroderma is an uncommon but important dermatological emergency, since the systemic effects are potentially fatal.

GENERAL SYMPTOMS AND SIGNS

Some features are common to all patients with erythroderma, no matter what the cause. It is twice as common in men and mainly affects the middle-aged and elderly. The condition often develops suddenly, particularly when associated with leukaemia or an eczema. A patchy erythema may rapidly spread to be universal within 12–48 hours and be accompanied by pyrexia, malaise and shivering. Scaling appears 2–6 days later, and at this stage the skin is hot, red, dry and obviously thickened. The patient experiences irritation and tightness of the skin and feels cold. The exfoliation of scales may be copious and continuous. Scalp and body hair is lost when erythroderma has been present for some weeks. The nails become thickened and may be shed. Pigmentary changes occur and, in those with a dark skin, hypopigmentation is seen. The picture is influenced by the patient's general condition and the underlying cause. The commonest causes of erythroderma are eczema, psoriasis and lymphoma (Table 1). Other dermatoses, including drug eruptions and pityriasis rubra pilaris, may also be implicated.

Eczema

Atopic eczema may become erythrodermic at any age. Erythroderma from eczema is most common in the elderly, in whom the eczema may be unclassified.

Table 1 **Causes of erythroderma and their relative frequencies**

Cause	%
Eczema (contact/atopic/seborrhoeic/ unclassified)	40%
Psoriasis	25%
Lymphoma/Sézary syndrome	15%
Drug eruption	10%
Pityriasis rubra pilaris/ichthyosiform erythroderma	1%
Other skin disease	1%
Unknown	8%

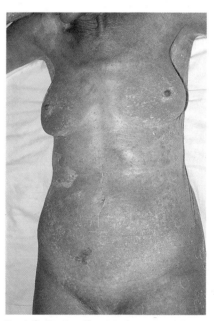

Fig. 1 **Erythrodermic psoriasis.**

Psoriasis

At first the eruption resembles conventional psoriasis, but when the exfoliative stage is reached, these specific features are lost (Fig. 1). The withdrawal of potent topical steroids or of systemic steroids, or an intercurrent drug eruption, can precipitate erythrodermic psoriasis. Sterile pinhead-sized pustules sometimes develop and the condition may progress to generalized pustular psoriasis (p. 27).

Lymphoma/Sézary syndrome

Early biopsies may not be specific and this may delay diagnosis, although universal erythroderma, infiltration of the skin and severe pruritus are helpful pointers (p. 85). Lymphadenopathy is often prominent, but the nodes are not always involved by lymphoma. Sézary syndrome occurs in elderly males and is characterized by the presence of abnormal T lymphocytes with large convoluted nuclei (Sézary cells) in the blood and skin (Fig. 2). Patients may be stable for a number of years then deteriorate rapidly.

Drug eruption

An acute drug eruption (p. 82), often of the toxic erythema or morbilliform type, may become erythrodermic (Fig. 3). Allopurinol, gold, isoniazid, PAS, phenytoin, sulphonamides and sulphonylureas are the commonest culprits.

Pityriasis rubra pilaris

Pityriasis rubra pilaris is a disorder of unknown aetiology which begins in adults with redness and scaling of the scalp and progresses to cover the limbs and trunk (Fig. 4). It is a follicle-based

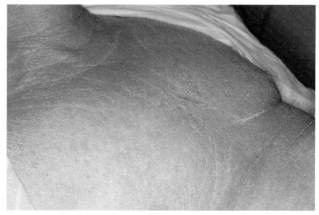

Fig. 2 **Erythroderma and infiltration of the skin due to the Sézary syndrome.**

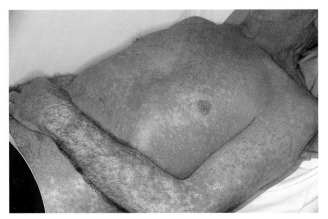

Fig. 3 **An erythrodermic reaction to an anti-inflammatory drug.**

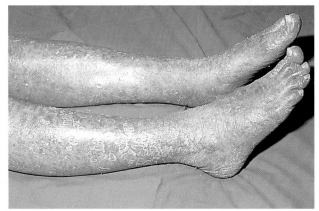

Fig. 4 **Pityriasis rubra pilaris affecting the legs.**

eruption and characteristically shows islands of sparing and a yellow keratotic thickening of the palms (Fig. 5). Treatment with retinoids will bring the eruption under control. Clearance occurs spontaneously in 1–3 years. A relapsing childhood type is reported.

Other dermatoses

Ichthyosiform erythroderma is a type of inherited ichthyosis (p. 86) which is present from birth or early infancy. Acute graft-versus-host disease and, very occasionally, severe scabies or extensive pemphigus can cause erythroderma.

In less than 10% of cases of erythroderma no cause is found. The possibility of a latent lymphoma must be considered.

COMPLICATIONS

Erythroderma is associated with profound physiological and metabolic changes (Table 2). Cardiac failure and hypothermia are risks, especially in the elderly, and cutaneous or respiratory infection may also occur. Oedema is almost invariable and cannot be regarded as a sign of heart failure. The pulse rate is always increased. Cardiac failure and infection are difficult to diagnose. Blood cultures are easily contaminated with skin microflora. Lymphadenopathy is common and does not necessarily signify lymphoma. In the pre-steroid era, erythroderma was fatal in one third of cases, largely due to cardiac failure or to infection.

MANAGEMENT

Inpatient treatment and skilled nursing care is mandatory. The patient is nursed in a comfortably warm room at a steady temperature (preferably

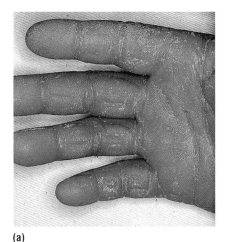

(a)

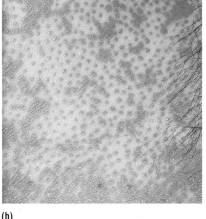

(b)

Fig. 5 **Pityriasis rubra pilaris.** (**a**) Yellowish hyperkeratosis of the palms. (**b**) Typical follicular lesions.

Table 2 **Pathophysiology of erythroderma**

Clinical complication	Pathophysiology
Cardiac failure	Increased cardiac output Increased plasma volume
Cutaneous oedema	Increased capillary permeability Increased plasma volume Hypoalbuminaemia
Hypoalbuminaemia	Increased plasma volume Protein loss in exfoliated scale Protein losing enteropathy
Dehydration	Increased transepidermal water loss Increased capillary permeability
Impaired temperature regulation	Excess heat loss Failure to sweat
Dermopathic lymphadenopathy	Cutaneous inflammation and infection

30–32°C), and the pulse, blood pressure, temperature and fluid balance are regularly monitored. An air-fluidized bed is sometimes used. Topical steroids and bland creams are a mainstay of local treatment and are often adequate. Systemic steroids are life-saving in severe cases. The maintenance of normal haemodynamics, attention to electrolyte equilibrium and adequate

nutritional support (particularly with regard to minimizing protein losses) are vital for severely ill patients. Cardiac failure and intercurrent infections are treated as necessary.

Erythroderma

- A rare but potentially fatal eruption often of sudden onset showing near universal skin involvement.
- Commonest causes: psoriasis, eczema and lymphoma.
- Characterized by red, oedematous, exfoliating skin.
- Complications include cardiac failure, hypothermia, infection and lymphadenopathy.
- Inpatient management and close supervision are required.
- Treatment consists initially of topical steroids and bland emollients. Systemic steroids and full supportive therapy may be needed in life-threatening cases.

PHOTODERMATOLOGY

PHOTODERMATOSES — IDIOPATHIC

POLYMORPHIC LIGHT ERUPTION

Polymorphic light eruption is a dermatosis of unknown aetiology characterized by papules, plaques and, sometimes, vesicles in light-exposed areas.

Clinical presentation

This is the commonest photodermatosis, and women are affected twice as frequently as men. Pruritic urticated papules, plaques and vesicles develop on light-exposed skin usually about 24 hours after sun exposure (Fig. 1). It starts in the spring and may persist throughout the summer. The degree of severity is variable.

Differential diagnosis and management

Photoallergic contact dermatitis, drug-induced photosensitivity and lupus erythematosus may need to be considered in diagnosis of polymorphic light eruption.

The first-line therapy is to use sunscreens and protective measures. A short course of PUVA in the late spring can 'harden' the skin so that the patient is able to have a disease-free summer.

ACTINIC RETICULOID/CHRONIC ACTINIC DERMATITIS

Chronic actinic dermatitis is a rare condition of unknown cause affecting middle-aged or elderly men who develop thick plaques of dermatitis on sun-exposed skin.

Histologically, the skin shows a dense lymphocytic infiltrate. Some of the lymphocytes may be atypical and suggest lymphoma (hence the name).

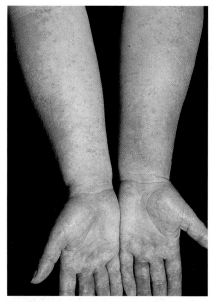

Fig. 1 **Polymorphic light eruption affecting the forearms.**

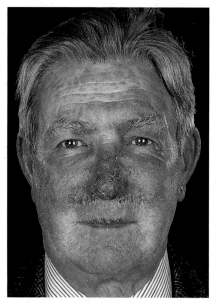

Fig. 2 **Chronic actinic dermatitis involving the light-exposed areas of the face.**

Clinical presentation

There is often a long history of a chronic contact dermatitis which evolves into a photodermatitis, or a photocontact dermatitis may have been present from the outset. Lichenified plaques of chronic dermatitis form on light-exposed sites and beyond, and are worse in the summer, although the eruption tends to become perennial (Fig. 2). The patients are sensitive to the UVA and UVB wavelengths and often to visible light as well. They may also have a contact or photocontact sensitivity to plant oleoresins (airborne allergens) or to cosmetic ingredients, although the relevance of this is uncertain.

Differential diagnosis and management

Airborne contact dermatitis or drug-induced photosensitivity may need to be considered, but normally there is little doubt about the diagnosis.

Light avoidance, sunscreens and topical steroids are used at first in the management of chronic actinic dermatitis. Subsequently, systemic steroids and azathioprine may be necessary.

SOLAR URTICARIA AND ACTINIC PRURIGO

Solar urticaria and actinic prurigo are rare conditions. In solar urticaria, wheals appear within minutes of sunlight exposure. Differentiation is required from erythropoietic protoporphyria (p. 43), especially in childhood. Actinic prurigo starts in childhood and is characterized by papules and excoriations mainly on sun-exposed sites.

PHOTODERMATOSES — OTHER CAUSES

GENETIC DISORDERS

Certain rare genetic disorders show photosensitivity. They may have chromosome instability (e.g. Bloom's syndrome) or defective DNA repair (e.g. xeroderma pigmentosum, p. 89).

METABOLIC DISORDERS

Porphyrias

Porphyrins are important in the formation of haemoglobin, myoglobin and cytochromes. The porphyrias are rare, mostly inherited, metabolic disorders in which deficiencies

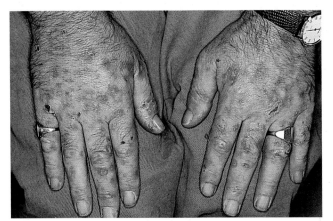

Fig. 3 Porphyria cutanea tarda. Changes can be seen on the dorsal aspects of the hands.

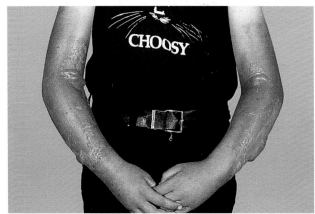

Fig. 4 Phytophotodermatitis to common rue. The patient had been gathering the plant in the bright sunlight and developed an extreme bullous reaction.

of enzymes in the porphyrin biosynthetic pathway lead to accumulations of intermediate metabolites (p. 80). The metabolites are detectable in the urine, faeces and blood, are toxic for the nervous system, and cause photosensitivity in the skin.

The main cutaneous porphyrias are:

- *Erythropoietic protoporphyria.* Autosomal dominant and starting in childhood, this is a red blistering eruption which leaves pitted scars on the nose and hands.
- *Porphyria cutanea tarda.* This is the commonest porphyria, seen mostly in male alcoholics with liver damage. Sun-induced subepidermal blisters on the face and hands (Fig. 3) leave fragile, scarred and hairy skin. Alcohol and aggravating drugs (e.g. oestrogens) are avoided. Venesection or low-dose chloroquine therapy may be used.
- *Variegate porphyria.* Autosomal dominant and common in South Africa. The skin signs are like porphyria cutanea tarda, but abdominal pain and neuropsychiatric symptoms resemble *acute intermittent porphyria*, which has no skin features.

Pellagra

Dietary deficiency of nicotinic acid may give a photosensitive dermatitis in association with diarrhoea and dementia.

DUE TO DRUGS OR CHEMICALS

Drug-induced

Several drugs may produce an eruption in light-exposed areas by either dose-dependent or allergic mechanisms. The morphology may be eczematous, blistering (e.g. nalidixic acid, p. 17), pigmented (e.g. amio-

Table 1 **Drugs causing photosensitivity**

ACE inhibitors	Nonsteroidal anti-inflammatories
Amiodarone	Phenothiazines
Ciprofloxacin	Protriptyline
Nalidixic acid	Tetracyclines
Nifedipine	Thiazides

darone, p. 83) or an exaggerated sunburn reaction. Rarely photo-onycholysis can occur (e.g. with tetracycline). Common photosensitizing drugs are shown in Table 1.

Topically applied chemicals

The commonest topical photosensitizers are coal tar and plant-derived pso-

ralens. Coal-tar products are used in the treatment of psoriasis and may photosensitize the patient's skin. Psoralens occur widely in plants and are found, for example, in carrot, celery, fennel, parsnip, common rue and giant hogweed. Phytophotodermatitis describes a photo-contact dermatitis which results from the local photosensitization of the skin through contact with psoralens from a plant (Fig. 4). In Berloque dermatitis, streaky pigmentation, often on the sides of the neck, results from the application of perfumes containing psoralens, usually Oil of Bergamot (p. 103).

DERMATOSES IMPROVED OR WORSENED BY SUNLIGHT

UV improves certain conditions (Table 2) and is used as a treatment either as natural sunlight, UVB or by PUVA. However, benefit is not observed in every case and, for example, a patient's psoriasis or atopic eczema can be made worse by UV. Psoriasis may even be precipitated by the sun. Several other conditions, listed in Table 2, are well recognized to be aggravated by the sun.

Table 2 **Dermatoses improved or aggravated by sunlight**

Improved	Worsened or provoked
Acne	Darier's disease
Atopic eczema	Herpes simplex
Mycosis fungoides	Lupus erythematosus
Parapsoriasis	Porphyrias
Pityriasis rosea	Rosacea
Psoriasis	Vitiligo

Photodermatology

- In normal skin, sunlight can cause tanning, sunburn, and, in time, photoageing (p. 100).
- The important idiopathic photodermatoses are: polymorphic light eruption, actinic reticuloid/chronic actinic dermatitis and solar urticaria.
- Dermatoses worsened by sunlight include Darier's disease, herpes simplex, LE, porphyria, rosacea and vitiligo.
- Dermatoses improved by sunlight include acne, atopic eczema, chronic superficial dermatitis (parapsoriasis), pityriasis rosea and psoriasis.
- Drugs which not infrequently cause photosensitivity include tetracyclines, phenothiazines, ACE inhibitors, nonsteroidal anti-inflammatories and thiazides.

BACTERIAL INFECTION — Staphylococcal and Streptococcal

The skin is a barrier to infection, but if its defences are penetrated or broken down, numerous microorganisms can cause disease (Table 1).

THE NORMAL SKIN MICROFLORA

Normal skin has a resident flora of usually harmless microorganisms, including bacteria, yeasts and mites. The bacteria are mostly staphylococci (e.g. *Staph. epidermidis*), micrococci, corynebacteria (diphtheroids) and propionibacteria. They cluster in the stratum corneum or hair follicles, and their number varies between individuals and between different sites on the body. Micrococci, for example, number 0.5 million per cm^2 in the axilla but only 60 per cm^2 on the forearm.

STAPHYLOCOCCAL INFECTIONS

About 20% of people intermittently carry *Staph. aureus* in the nose, axilla or perineum. Staphylococci can infect the skin directly or secondarily, as in eczema or psoriasis.

IMPETIGO

Impetigo is a superficial skin infection due either to staphylococci or streptococci, or both.

Clinical presentation

Impetigo is now relatively uncommon in the UK, due mainly to improved social conditions. It generally occurs in children and presents as thin-walled easily ruptured blisters, often on the face, which leave areas of yellow crusted exudate (Fig. 1). Lesions spread rapidly and are contagious. A bullous form, with blisters 1–2 cm in diameter, is seen in all ages and affects the face or extremities. Atopic eczema, scabies, herpes simplex and lice infestation may all become impetiginized. Impetigo can be confused with herpes simplex or a fungal infection.

Management

Most localized cases respond to the removal of the crusts with saline soaks and the application of a topical antibiotic (e.g. neomycin, chlortetracycline, mupirocin or fusidic acid). Systemic erythromycin or flucloxacillin are given for widespread infection. Impetigo caused by *Strep. pyogenes* may result in glomerulonephritis, a serious complication. Oral phenoxymethylpenicillin (penicillin V) is prescribed where infection with nephritogenic streptococci is suspected.

ECTHYMA

Ecthyma is characterized by circumscribed, ulcerated and crusted infected lesions which heal with scarring. An insect bite or neglected minor injury may become infected with staphylococci or streptococci. Ecthyma mostly occurs on the legs (Fig. 2) and may be seen in drug addicts or debilitated patients. Treatment is with systemic and topical antibiotics.

FOLLICULITIS AND RELATED CONDITIONS

Infection can affect hair follicles. *Folliculitis* is an acute pustular infection of multiple hair follicles, a *furuncle* is an acute abscess formation in adjacent hair follicles, and a *carbuncle* is a deep abscess formed in a group of follicles giving a painful suppurating mass.

Clinical presentation

Follicular pustules are seen in hair-bearing areas, e.g. the legs or face. In men, folliculitis may affect the beard area (sycosis barbae). In women, it may occur on the legs after hair removal by shaving or waxing. *Staph. aureus* is usually but not invariably responsible. A Gram-negative folliculitis (e.g. with pseudomonas) may occur with prolonged antibiotic treatment for acne. *Pityrosporum folliculitis* is a separate condition due to a commensal yeast (p. 34).

Furuncles (boils) present as tender red pustules which suppurate and heal with scarring. They often occur on the

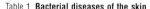
Table 1 **Bacterial diseases of the skin**

Organism	Infection
Commensals	Erythrasma, pitted keratolysis, trichomycosis axillaris
Staphylococcal	Impetigo, ecthyma, folliculitis, secondary infection
Streptococcal	Erysipelas, cellulitis, impetigo, ecthyma, necrotizing fasciitis
Gram-negative	Secondary infection, folliculitis, cellulitis
Mycobacterial	TB (lupus vulgaris, warty tuberculosis, scrofuloderma), fish tank granuloma, Buruli ulcer, leprosy
Spirochaetal	Syphilis (primary, secondary, etc), Lyme disease (erythema chronicum migrans)
Neisseria	Gonorrhoea (pustules), meningococcaemia (purpura)
Others	Anthrax (pustule), erysipeloid (pustule)

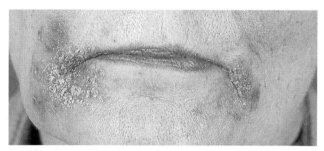
Fig. 1 **Impetigo of the face due to *Staph. aureus*.**

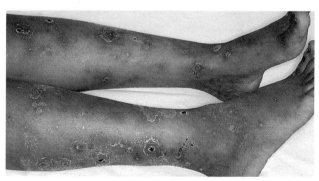
Fig. 2 **Ecthyma, due to a streptococcus, affecting the lower legs.**

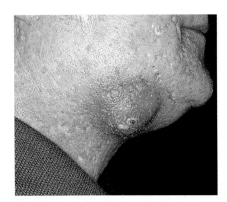

Fig. 3 **A carbuncle.** This required surgical drainage. The patient had had previous staphylococcal infection.

face, neck, scalp, axillae and perineum. Some patients have recurrent staphylococcal boils of the axillae or perineum. Large suppurating carbuncles (Fig. 3) due to *Staph. aureus* may cause systemic upset.

Management

Swabs for bacterial culture are taken from the lesion and from carrier sites, e.g. the nose, axilla and groin. Obesity, diabetes mellitus and occlusion from clothing are predisposing factors. Acute staphylococcal infections are treated with antibiotics both systemic (e.g. flucloxacillin or erythromycin) and topical (e.g. neomycin, fusidic acid or mupirocin). Chronic and recurrent cases are more difficult. Carrier sites need treatment with a topical antibiotic (e.g. mupirocin). General measures such as improved hygiene, regular bathing or showering, the use of antiseptics in the bath and on the skin (e.g. chlorhexidine) can help, but courses of oral antibiotics may be needed. Carbuncles often need prompt surgical drainage. An infrequent complication is thrombosis in the cavernous sinus, associated with facial infection.

STAPHYLOCOCCAL SCALDED SKIN SYNDROME

Staphylococcal scalded skin syndrome is an acute toxic illness, usually of infants, characterized by shedding of sheets of skin and infection with phage type 71 staphylococci. The condition may follow impetigo. Large epidermal sheets are shed, resembling a scald, leaving denuded erythematous areas. The staphylococci release an exotoxin which causes the epidermis to split. A related condition in adults is mostly drug-induced (p. 83).

Although a serious condition, requiring inpatient treatment, the prognosis is good when systemic flucloxacillin or erythromycin are prescribed.

STREPTOCOCCAL INFECTIONS

Strep. pyogenes, the principal human skin pathogen, is occasionally found in the throat and may persist after an infection. It is sometimes carried in the nose and can contaminate and colonize damaged skin.

ERYSIPELAS

Erysipelas is an acute infection of the dermis by *Strep. pyogenes*. It shows well-demarcated erythema, oedema and tenderness.

Clinical presentation

The skin lesions may be preceeded by fever, malaise and 'flu-like' symptoms. Erysipelas usually affects the face (where it may be bilateral) or the lower leg, and appears as a painful red swelling (Fig. 4). The lesion has a well-defined edge and may blister. The streptococci usually gain entry to the skin via a fissure, e.g. behind the ear, or associated with tinea pedis between the toes.

Differential diagnosis and complications

On the face, erysipelas may be confused with angioedema or allergic contact dermatitis, but the condition is usually distinguished as it causes tenderness and systemic upset. Recurrent attacks in the same place can result in lymphoedema due to lymphatic damage. A fatal streptococcal septicaemia can occur in debilitated patients. Guttate psoriasis (p. 27)

and acute glomerulonephritis may follow a streptococcal infection.

Management

A good response is usually seen with prompt treatment. Topical therapy is inappropriate, and penicillin should be prescribed. *Strep. pyogenes* is nearly always sensitive. Parenteral treatment is needed at first for a severe infection, usually with benzylpenicillin for 2 or so days. Oral penicillin V can then be given for 7–14 days. In less severe cases, penicillin V is adequate. Erythromycin is used if there is penicillin allergy. Recurrent

erysipelas, i.e. more than two episodes at one site, requires prophylactic long-term penicillin V (250 mg once or twice a day), with attention to hygiene at potential portals of entry.

NECROTIZING FASCIITIS

Necrotizing fasciitis is an acute and serious infection. It usually occurs in otherwise healthy subjects after minor trauma. An ill-defined erythema, often on the leg and associated with a high fever, rapidly becomes necrotic. Early surgical debridement and systemic antibiotics are essential.

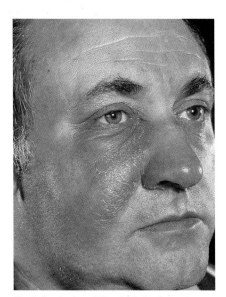

Fig. 4 **Erysipelas of the right cheek due to a streptococcal infection.**

Staphylococcal and streptococcal infections

- *Normal skin microflora* includes staphylococci, micrococci, corynebacteria and propionibacteria, and may number 0.5 million per cm^2.
- *Staphylococcal infection* of the skin may be primary, e.g. impetigo, ecthyma or folliculitis, or secondary, e.g. superinfection of eczema, psoriasis or leg ulcers.
- *Streptococcal infections* may also be primary, e.g. erysipelas or cellulitis, or secondary, e.g. infection of dermatoses or leg ulcers.

OTHER BACTERIAL INFECTIONS

DISEASES DUE TO COMMENSAL OVERGROWTH

Sometimes 'normal' commensals can result in disease. Among the most common are:

- *Erythrasma*. A dry, reddish-brown, slightly scaly and usually asymptomatic eruption affecting the body folds (Fig. 1). It fluoresces coral-pink with Wood's light, due to the production of porphyrins by the corynebacteria. Imidazole creams, topical fusidic acid or oral erythromycin are effective.
- *Trichomycosis axillaris*. Overgrowths of corynebacteria form yellow concretions on axillary hair. Topical antimicrobials usually effect a cure.
- *Pitted keratolysis*. Overgrowth of micrococci, which digest keratin, occurs with occluding footwear and

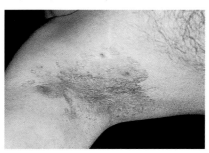

Fig. 1 **Erythrasma affecting the axilla.** This was due to overgrowth of corynebacteria.

sweaty feet (Fig. 2). Malodorous pitted erosions and depressed, discoloured areas result. Better hygiene, topical neomycin, or soaks with 0.01% aqueous potassium permanganate or 3% aqueous formaldehyde usually help.

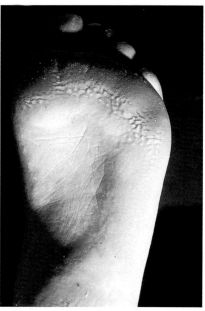

Fig. 2 **Pitted keratolysis, due to a micrococcus.**

MYCOBACTERIAL INFECTIONS

Mycobacterium tuberculosis and *M. leprae* (p. 56) are the most important mycobacteria in human disease, although other species can cause infections. In many Western countries, TB recently has shown a resurgence, in part related to increasing numbers of patients with HIV infection. In addition, it is a major problem in the Third World. TB can produce a number of cutaneous manifestations (Table 1).

Table 1 **Skin manifestations of tuberculosis**

Lupus vulgaris
Tuberculides
Scrofuloderma
Warty tuberculosis

LUPUS VULGARIS

Lupus vulgaris is characterized by reddish-brown plaques, often on the head or neck. It is the commonest *M. tuberculosis* skin infection.

Clinical presentation

Lupus vulgaris follows primary inoculation and develops in individuals with some immunity. It begins as painless reddish-brown nodules which slowly enlarge to form a plaque (Fig. 3), leaving scarring and sometimes

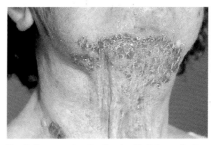

Fig. 3 **Lupus vulgaris, due to *M. tuberculosis*.**

destruction of deeper tissues such as cartilage. Presentation in the elderly often is due to reactivation of pre-existing inadequately treated disease.

Differential diagnosis and complications

Papules of lupus vulgaris typically show an 'apple-jelly' colour when compressed with a glass slide (diascopy). A biopsy will reveal tuberculoid granulomata with a few bacilli. The Mantoux test is positive. Sometimes it is necessary to consider:

- morphoeic basal cell carcinoma
- sarcoidosis
- discoid lupus erythematosus.

Squamous cell carcinoma may develop in long-standing scarred lesions. The presence of *M. tuberculosis* somewhere in the body can induce cutaneous reactions ('tuberculides'). *Erythema nodosum* (p. 79) is the best-known example. Another is *erythema induratum* which occurs as painful ulcerating nodules on the lower legs of women and is thought to be a hypersensitivity response to TB.

Management

At least three drugs (normally rifampicin, isoniazid and pyrazinamide, possibly with either ethambutol or streptomycin) are given for the initial 8 weeks. After this it is usual to continue with isoniazid and rifampicin, under close supervision, to complete a 6–9 month course. The duration of treatment depends to some extent on response.

SCROFULODERMA

A tuberculous lymph node or joint can directly involve the overlying skin, often on the neck. Fistulae and scarring result.

WARTY TUBERCULOSIS

A warty plaque, often on the hands, knees or buttock, results from inoculation of the TB bacillus into the skin of someone with immunity from previous infection. It is rare in Western countries but is the commonest form of cutaneous TB in the Third World.

OTHER CUTANEOUS MYCOBACTERIAL INFECTIONS

Fish tank granuloma

Typically this is a reddish, slightly scaly plaque on the hand or arm of someone who keeps tropical fish. It is due to *M. marinum* which infects fish, and is also found in swimming pools.

Buruli ulcer

In tropical zones, *M. ulcerans* — acquired from vegetation or water after trauma — produces a painless erythematous nodule usually on the leg or forearm. The nodule becomes necrotic and ulceration results.

M. avium complex infection is seen in patients with AIDS (p. 52).

SPIROCHAETAL INFECTIONS

Spirochaetes are thin, spiral and motile organisms. Syphilis (p. 112), due to *Treponema pallidum*, is the best-known spirochaetal disease, but other spirochaetes, e.g. *Borrelia burgdorferi*, can be pathogenic.

NON-VENEREAL TREPONEMAL INFECTIONS

Non-venereal treponemal infections are endemic in tropical and subtropical areas where people live in conditions of extreme poverty. They are caused by spirochaetes which are very similar to *Treponema pallidum*. Serological tests for syphilis are posi-tive. All three diseases discussed below respond to penicillin.

- *Yaws* occurs in central Africa, central America and southeast Asia. In children the treponeme enters the skin through an abrasion, and after a few weeks results in an ulcerated papilloma which heals with scarring. Secondary lesions follow, and, in the late stage, bone deformities develop.
- *Bejel* (endemic syphilis), found in the middle east, is similar to yaws but starts around the mouth. It is transmitted on drinking cups and may spread within families.
- *Pinta* is confined to central and south America, It results in hyper-keratoses over extensor aspects of joints with both hypo- and hyperpigmentation.

LYME DISEASE

Lyme disease is a cutaneous and systemic infection caused by the spirochaete *Borrelia burgdorferi* and spread by tick-bite. Most cases have been reported in the USA and Europe. At the site of the tick bite, usually a limb, a slowly expanding erythematous ring (erythema chronicum

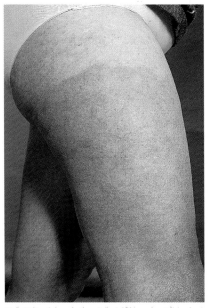

Fig. 4 **Erythema chronicum migrans of Lyme disease.**

migrans) develops (Fig. 4). Arthritis, neurological and cardiac disease may follow. A response to penicillin or tetracycline is usual.

FURTHER BACTERIAL INFECTIONS

ANTHRAX

A haemorrhagic bulla, associated with oedema and fever, forms at the site of inoculation of the skin with *Bacillus anthracis*, usually from contaminated animal products. It is now rare. Penicillin is curative.

GRAM-NEGATIVE INFECTIONS

Bacilli such as *Pseudomonas aeruginosa* can infect skin wounds, notably leg ulcers. They may also cause folliculitis and cellulitis.

CELLULITIS

Cellulitis is an infection of the subcutaneous tissues. It is often due to streptococci, but is deeper and more extensive than erysipelas. The cardinal features are swelling, redness and local pain with systemic upset and fever. The leg is often affected (Fig. 5). The organism may gain entry through fissures between the toes or via a leg ulcer. Lymphangitis is common, and lymphatic damage may result. Hospital admission is usually indicated, particularly if the leg is involved. Antistreptococcal antibiotics are given for straight-forward cases. However, a broad spectrum antibiotic is prescribed for cellulitis complicating a leg ulcer, since a selection of organisms may be responsible. Blood cultures and ulcer swabs may give some guidance.

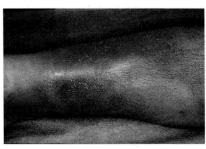

Fig. 5 **Cellulitis affecting the lower leg.**

> **Other bacterial infections**
>
> - Overgrowth of commensal organisms can result in minor skin 'disease'.
> - Cutaneous mycobacterial infection is mainly due to *M. tuberculosis*, but occasionally 'atypical' mycobacteria such as *M. marinum*, cause disease.
> - Non-venereal treponematoses, yaws, pinta and bejel, are important diseases in the Third World.
> - Lyme disease is a tick-transmitted infection with *Borrelia burgdorferi;* the skin signs often are associated with systemic disease.
> - Cellulitis often affects the leg and frequently is caused by streptococci, though other organisms may be involved.

VIRAL INFECTIONS — Warts and Other Viral Infections

Unlike bacteria and yeasts, viruses are not thought to exist on the skin surface as commensals. However, studies in patients with viral warts have shown viral DNA in epidermal cells of seemingly normal skin next to warty areas.

VIRAL WARTS

Warts (verrucae) are common and benign cutaneous tumours due to infection of epidermal cells with human papilloma virus.

Aetiopathogenesis and pathology

Over 50 subtypes of DNA human papilloma virus (HPV) have been identified. The virus infects by direct inoculation and is caught by touch, sexual contact or at the swimming baths. Certain HPV subtypes are associated with specific clinical lesions, e.g. type 2 with common hand warts, types 1 and 4 with plantar warts, types 6, 11, 16 and 18 with genital warts. Genital HPV subtypes cause cytological dysplasia of the cervix which may be precancerous. Immunosuppressed individuals, such as those with renal transplants, are particularly susceptible to viral warts (p. 53). The epidermis is thickened and hyperkeratotic. Keratinocytes in the granular layer are vacuolated due to being infected with the wart virus.

Clinical presentation

Certain clinical patterns are well recognized:

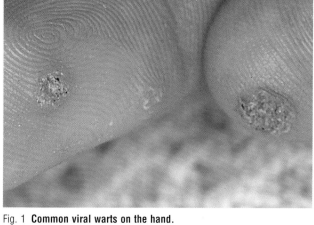

Fig. 1 **Common viral warts on the hand.**

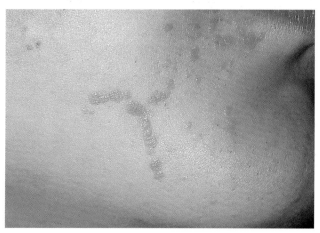

Fig. 2 **Plane viral warts on the face.**

- *Common warts*. These present as dome-shaped papules or nodules with a papilliferous surface. They are usually multiple, and are commonest on the hands (Fig. 1) or feet in children but also affect the face and genitalia. Their surface interrupts skin lines. Some facial warts are 'filiform' with fine digit-like projections.
- *Plane warts*. These are smooth flat-topped papules, often slightly brown in colour, and commonest on the face (Fig. 2) and dorsal aspects of the hands. They are usually multiple and resist treatment, but eventually resolve spontaneously, often after becoming inflamed. They can show the Koebner phenomenon.
- *Plantar warts*. These are seen in children and adolescents on the soles of the feet; pressure causes them to grow into the dermis. They are painful and covered by callus, which, when pared, reveals dark punctate spots (thrombosed capillaries). Mosaic warts are plaques on the soles which comprise multiple individual warts.
- *Genital warts*. In males these affect the penis, and in homosexuals, the perianal area. In females, the vulva, perineum and vagina may be involved (Fig. 3). The warts may be small, or may coalesce into large cauliflower-like 'condylomata acuminata'. Proctoscopy (if perianal warts are present) and colposcopy (for female genital warts) are needed to identify and treat any rectal or cervical warts because of the risk of neoplastic change. Sexual partners need to be examined.

Differential diagnosis and complications

The diagnosis of viral warts is usually obvious. Occasionally, a corn on the sole or hand, or molluscum contagiosum elsewhere, are confused. With viral warts, under the fingernails and toenails, it is important to consider amelanotic malignant melanoma, periungual fibroma (of tuberous sclerosis, p. 88) and bony subungual exostosis. Genital warts may resemble the condyloma lata of secondary syphilis. HPV types 16 and 18 in genital warts carry a risk of malignant change. HPV infections in renal transplant patients have been linked with skin cancers.

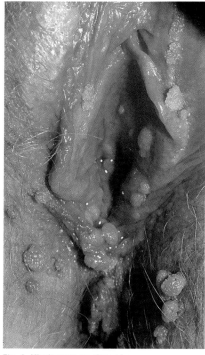

Fig. 3 **Viral warts on the vulva.**

Management

In children, 30–50% of common warts disappear spontaneously within 6 months. Hand and foot warts should be pared by a scalpel or using a pumice stone. This gets rid of keratotic skin and allows easier treatment. Table 1 shows the available treatments. Immunosuppressed patients, especially those with renal transplants, are prone to wart infections. They need special management and should be inspected and treated for warts before being given their grafts.

OTHER VIRAL INFECTIONS

Other viral infections include molluscum contagiosum, orf, HIV (p. 52) and those in Table 2.

Molluscum contagiosum

Molluscum contagiosum are discrete pearly-pink umbilicated papules which are caused by a DNA pox virus. Mollusca mainly affect children or young adults. Spread is by contact, including sexual transmission or on towels. The dome-shaped papule, a few mm in diameter, has a punctum and if squeezed, releases a cheesy material. The lesions are usually multiple and grouped, and are commonest on the face, neck and trunk (Fig. 4). Isolated ones may go unrecognized. Untreated, they may persist for several months.

In the adult or older child, removal is by expressing the contents with forceps, curettage under local anaesthesia or cryotherapy. These measures are poorly tolerated in young children, and the best approach is to instruct the parents to squeeze out the 'ripe' lesions after the child has bathed.

Orf

Orf usually occurs as a solitary, rapidly growing papule, often on the hand.

Table 1 **Treatments for viral warts**

Modality	Details	Indication	Contraindications/side effects
Topical	Salicylic and lactic acids (e.g. Salactol, Duofilm, Salatac)	Hand and foot warts	Facial/anogenital warts, atopic eczema
	Glutaraldehyde (e.g. Glutarol)	Hand and foot warts	Facial/anogenital warts, atopic eczema
	Formaldehyde (5% aqueous)	Foot warts	Facial/anogenital warts, atopic eczema
	Podophyllin (15%) paint	Genital warts	Pregnancy (teratogenic)
Cryotherapy	Applied every 3-4 weeks	Hand and foot, genital warts	May cause blistering
Curettage and cautery	Local anaesthetic (or general anaesthetic if large)	Solitary filiform warts, especially on face. Large perineal warts	Not recommended for hand or foot warts as scars may result; warts may recur
Other	Intralesional bleomycin	Resistant hand/foot warts	Procedure can be painful
	Laser surgery	Any type of wart	Specialized treatment at present
	Interferon	Resistant (genital) warts	Systemic side effects

Table 2 **Other viral infections**

Disorder	Cause	Clinical presentation	Course and management
Fifth disease (erythema infectiosum)	Parvovirus B19	Slapped cheek sign, lace-like erythema over shoulders, sometimes arthralgia	Small outbreaks affect children aged 3–12 years; fades in 11 days; treatment unnecessary
Gianotti-Crosti syndrome	Hepatitis B and other viruses	Small red lichenoid papules on face, buttocks and extremities	Affects young children (peak 1–6 y); clears in about 3 weeks
Hand, foot and mouth disease	Coxsackie A16	Oral blisters/ulcers, red-edged vesicles on hands/feet, mild fever	Epidemics in young children; fades in 1 week; no treatment needed
Kawasaki disease	Unknown organism	Generalized erythema, peeling of hands/feet, strawberry tongue, fever, myocarditis, lymphadenopathy, coronary artery aneurysms	Affects young children; usually resolves in 2 weeks; investigate for cardiac involvement
Measles	RNA virus	Koplik's spots on buccal mucosa, morbilliform rash	Rash fades after the 6–10th day

The orf pox virus is endemic in sheep and causes a pustular eruption around the muzzle area. Human infection is well recognized in country regions and occurs in shepherds, veterinary surgeons and, typically, the farmer's wife who has been bottle-feeding a lamb.

A solitary red papule appears, usually on a finger, after an incubation period of about 6 days (Fig. 5). It grows rapidly to 1 cm or so in size, evolving into a painful purple pustule which often has a necrotic umbilicated centre. Erythema multiforme (p. 78) and lymphangitis are complications.

Spontaneous resolution takes 2–4 weeks. Secondary infection requires a topical or systemic antibiotic.

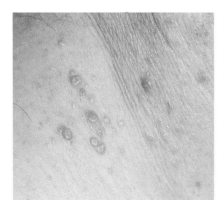

Fig. 4 **Molluscum contagiosum on the neck.**

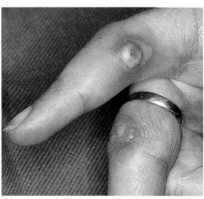

Fig. 5 **Orf on the fingers of a farmer's wife.**

Warts and other viral conditions

Viral warts
- Hand and foot warts are common and often disappear spontaneously.
- Try wart paints for hand and foot warts before proceeding to cryotherapy.
- Genital warts generally need cryotherapy.

Molluscum contagiosum
- Caused by a pox virus. Treated by expressing or cryotherapy.

Orf
- Found in rural areas.
- Diagnosis is usually obvious, but treat secondary infection and watch for erythema multiforme.

VIRAL INFECTIONS — Herpes Simplex and Herpes Zoster

HERPES SIMPLEX

Herpes simplex is a very common acute, self-limiting vesicular eruption due to infection with *Herpesvirus hominis*.

Aetiopathogenesis and pathology

Herpes simplex virus is highly contagious and is spread by direct contact with infected individuals. The virus penetrates the epidermis or mucous membrane epithelium and replicates within the epithelial cells. After the primary infection, the latent non-replicating virus resides mainly within the dorsal root ganglion, from whence it can reactivate, invade the skin and cause recrudescent lesions. There are two types of herpes simplex virus. *Type 1* disease is usually facial or non-genital, and *type 2* lesions are commonly genital, although this distinction is not absolute. The pathological changes of epidermal cell destruction by the herpes virus result in intra-epidermal vesicles and multi-nucleate giant cells. Infected cells may show intranuclear inclusions.

Clinical presentation

Type 1 primary infection usually occurs in childhood and is often sub-clinical. Acute gingivostomatitis is a common presentation in those with symptoms. Vesicles on the lips and mucous membranes quickly erode and are painful. Sometimes the cornea is involved. The illness is often accompanied by fever, malaise and local lymphadenopathy and lasts about 2 weeks.

Herpetic whitlow is another presentation (Fig. 1). A painful vesicle or pustule is found on a finger in, for example, a nurse or dentist attending a patient secreting the virus. Similar direct inoculation is sometimes seen in sportsmen such as wrestlers ('herpes gladiatorum').

Type 2 primary infection is normally seen after sexual contact in young adults, who develop acute vulvovaginitis, penile or perianal lesions. Culture-positive genital herpes simplex in a pregnant woman at the time of delivery is an indication for caesarean section, as neonatal infection can be fatal.

Recurrence is a hallmark of herpes simplex infection, and occurs at a similar site each time, usually on the lips, face (Fig. 2) or genitals (Fig. 3). Rarely, herpes simplex may appear in a zosteriform dermatomal distribution. The outbreak of groups of vesicles is often preceded for a few hours, by tingling or burning. Crusts form within 24–48 hours, and the infection fades after a week. Attacks may be precipitated by respiratory infection

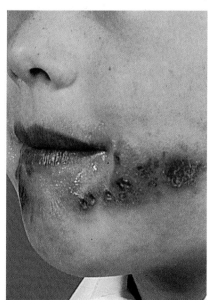

Fig. 2 **Herpes simplex on the cheek of a child.**

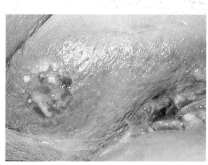

Fig. 3 **Genital lesions of recurrent herpes simplex.**

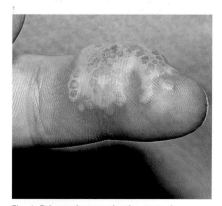

Fig. 1 **Primary herpes simplex occurring as a herpetic whitlow on a finger.**

(hence 'cold' sore), sunlight or local trauma.

Differential diagnosis

Occasionally herpes simplex can be confused with impetigo, but in recrudescent disease the recurrent nature usually indicates the diagnosis. If necessary, the virus can be cultured or detected by an immunofluorescent test.

Complications

Complications are infrequent but can be serious. They include:

- *Secondary bacterial infection.* This is usually due to *Staph. aureus.*
- *Eczema herpeticum.* Widespread herpes simplex infection is a serious and potentially fatal complication seen in patients with atopic eczema (p. 33) or Darier's disease (p. 87).
- *Disseminated herpes simplex.* Widespread herpetic vesicles may occur in the newborn or in immunosuppressed patients.
- *Chronic herpes simplex.* Atypical and chronic lesions may be seen in patients with HIV infection.
- *Herpes encephalitis.* This is a serious complication of herpes simplex, not always accompanied by skin lesions.
- *Carcinoma of the cervix.* This is more common in women with serological evidence of infection with Type II herpes simplex, which may be a predisposing factor.
- *Erythema multiforme.* Herpes simplex infection is the most common cause of recurrent erythema multiforme (p. 78).

Management

Mild herpetic lesions may not require any medication. The treatment of choice for recurrent mild facial or genital herpes simplex is aciclovir (Zovirax) cream (applied 5 times a day for 5 days), which reduces the length of the attack and the duration of viral shedding, and should preferably be started at the first indication of a recrudescence. More severe episodes warrant oral treatment with aciclovir (200 mg 5 times a day for 5 days) which shortens the attack. Long-term oral administration is useful in those with frequent recurrent attacks. Intravenous aciclovir may be life-saving in the immunosuppressed and in infants with eczema herpeticum. Genital herpes simplex can also be treated with famciclovir (p. 106). In those with genital herpes simplex, barrier contraception methods are advisable during intercourse, and intercourse should be avoided during symptomatic episodes.

HERPES ZOSTER

Herpes zoster (shingles) is an acute, self-limiting, vesicular eruption occurring in a dermatomal distribution; it is caused by a recrudescence of *Varicella zoster* virus.

Aetiopathogenesis and pathology

Herpes zoster nearly always occurs in subjects who have previously had varicella (chickenpox). The virus lies dormant in the sensory root ganglion of the spinal cord, but when reactivated, the virus replicates and migrates along the nerve to the skin, producing pain and ultimately inducing the cutaneous lesions of shingles. A viraemia is frequent, and disseminated involvement may be seen. The pathological changes are identical to those of herpes simplex.

Clinical presentation

Pain, tenderness or paraesthesia in the dermatome may precede the eruption by 3–5 days. Erythema and grouped vesicles follow, scattered within the dermatomal area (Fig. 4). The vesicles become pustular and then form crusts which separate in 2–3 weeks to leave scarring. Secondary bacterial infection may occur. Herpes zoster is normally unilateral and may involve adjacent dermatomes. The thoracic dermatomes are affected in 50% of cases and, in the elderly, involvement of the ophthalmic division of the trigeminal nerve is particularly common (Fig. 5). Two-thirds of patients with herpes zoster are over 50 years of age, and it is uncommon in children. The lesions shed virus, and contacts with no previous exposure may develop chickenpox.

Some scattering of vesicles outwith the dermatomal distribution is not uncommon, but disseminated or unusually haemorrhagic vesicles raise the possibility of immunosuppression or underlying malignancy. Local lymphadenopathy is usual, as is sensory disturbance of varying degree, including pain, numbness and paraesthesia. Shingles is recurrent in 5% of cases.

Differential diagnosis

The prodromal pain of herpes zoster can mimic cardiac or pleural pain, or an acute abdominal emergency. Once the eruption has appeared, the diagnosis is usually obvious, although herpes simplex may infrequently occur in a dermatomal fashion. Viral culture is sometimes needed.

Complications

Serious complications may occur in herpes zoster. These include:

- *Ophthalmic disease.* Corneal ulcers and scarring may result from shingles of the first trigeminal division. Ophthalmological assistance is mandatory.
- *Motor palsy.* Rarely, the viral involvement may spread from the posterior horn of the spinal cord to the anterior horn, and result in a motor disorder. Cranial nerve

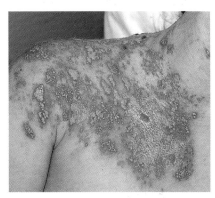

Fig. 4 **Herpes zoster of the C4 dermatome.**

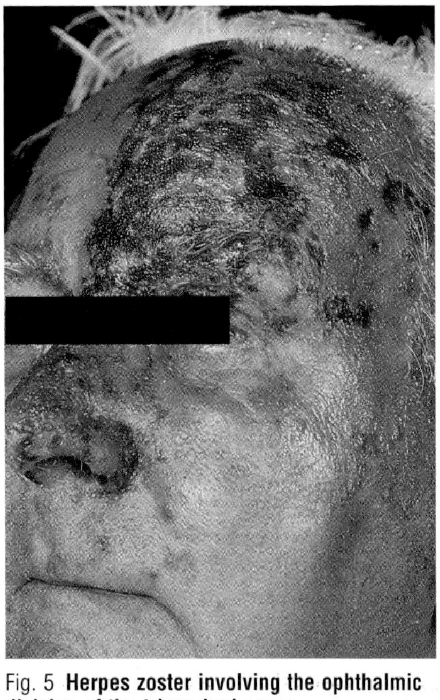

palsies or paralysis of the diaphragm or other muscle groups may occur.
- *Disseminated herpes zoster.* Immunosuppressed subjects, and patients with Hodgkin's disease especially, can develop confluent haemorrhagic involvement which spreads and may become necrotic or gangrenous. Varicella pneumonia or encephalitis are potentially fatal.
- *Post-herpetic neuralgia.* Neuralgia is infrequent in patients under 40 years but is found in a third of those over 60 years. The pain subsides in the majority within 12 months.

Management

In mild shingles, treatment is symptomatic, with rest, analgesia and bland drying preparations such as calamine lotion. Secondary bacterial infection may require a topical antiseptic or antibiotic. More severe cases may be treated, if seen within 48 hours of onset, with oral aciclovir (800 mg 5 times per day for 7 days) or famciclovir (p. 106) which promote resolution, reduce the viral shedding time and may reduce post-herpetic neuralgia. Immunosuppressed patients often require intravenous aciclovir or famciclovir. Oral prednisolone, given early in the course of herpes zoster for 14 days, reduces the incidence of post-herpetic neuralgia, but must not be used if the patient is immunosuppressed. Post-herpetic neuralgia may respond to topical capsaicin (p. 106).

Fig. 5 **Herpes zoster involving the ophthalmic division of the trigeminal nerve.**

Herpes simplex and herpes zoster

Herpes simplex
- Type 1 infection: usually orofacial, childhood onset.
- Type 2 infection: mostly genital, adult onset.
- Characterized by recurrent bouts at the same locus.
- Aciclovir is an effective treatment.

Herpes zoster
- Recrudescence of dormant *Varicella zoster* virus.
- Dermatomal, especially thoracic and trigeminal distributions.
- Neuralgia may complicate, mainly in the elderly.
- Dissemination suggests underlying immunosuppression.

HIV DISEASE AND IMMUNODEFICIENCY SYNDROMES

Immunodeficiency results from absence or failure of one or more elements of the immune system. It may be acquired, e.g. AIDS, or inherited, e.g. chronic mucocutaneous candidiasis.

HUMAN IMMUNODEFICIENCY VIRUS (HIV) DISEASE

Infection with HIV is a progressive process which mostly leads to the development of acquired immune deficiency syndrome (AIDS).

AETIOPATHOGENESIS

HIV1 and HIV2 (the latter mainly found in West Africa) are retroviruses containing reverse transcriptase which allows incorporation of the virus into a cell's DNA. The virus infects and depletes helper/inducer CD4 T-lymphocytes, leading to loss of cell-mediated immunity and opportunistic infection, e.g. with *Pneumocystis carinii*, mycobacteria or cryptococci. HIV is spread by infected body fluids e.g. blood or semen. High-risk groups for HIV infection include male homosexuals, intravenous drug users and haemophiliacs who have received infected blood products.

CLINICAL PRESENTATION

The acute infection may be symptomless but, in 50% of cases, seroconversion is accompanied by a glandular fever-like illness with a maculopapular eruption on the trunk. HIV infection may be asymptomatic for several years although most infected individuals will eventually develop symptoms. In the early stages of symptomatic infection, skin changes, fatigue, weight loss, generalized lymphadenopathy, diarrhoea and fever are present without the opportunistic infections which define AIDS. Opportunistic organisms include the ubiquitous *Mycobacterium avium* complex and *Cryptococcus neoformans,* and toxoplasmosis and cytomegalovirus.

As the disease progresses, the number of CD4+ lymphocytes falls and, when the blood count is below 50 cells/μL in the late phase of HIV infection (AIDS), *M. avium* complex infection, lymphoma and encephalopathy may develop. The mean latent period

Table 1 **Skin signs and the progressive stages of HIV infection**

Stage	Primary phase	Early phase (asymptomatic)	Intermediate (AIDS-related complex)	Late phase (AIDS)
Skin signs	Transient maculopapular eruption on trunk	Hypersensitivity reactions, onset or worsening of eczemas, psoriasis or folliculitis, wart virus and fungal infections	Herpes zoster, eczemas worsen, candidiasis, Kaposi's sarcoma	Candidiasis, opportunistic infections, Kaposi's sarcoma, lymphoma

between infection and the development of AIDS is 10 years. Skin signs include (Table 1):

- *Dry skin*: Skin dryness, often with asteatotic eczema, and seborrhoeic dermatitis (Fig. 1), are common and early findings. Their severity increases as the disease advances.
- *Fungal and papilloma virus infections*: Tinea infections, and perianal and common viral warts, are seen in early disease.
- *Acne and folliculitis*: These worsen in early and mid-stage disease.
- *Other infections*: Oral candidiasis, oral hairy leukoplakia (thought to be due to proliferation of Epstein-Barr virus: Fig. 2), and infection with herpes simplex, herpes zoster, molluscum contagiosum and *Staphylococcus aureus* are increased in advanced disease.
- *Other dermatoses*: Drug eruptions, hyperpigmentation and basal cell carcinomas are more common, psoriasis can get worse and syphilis may coexist.
- *Kaposi's sarcoma*: Kaposi's sarcoma is a multicentric tumour of vascular endothelium seen in a third of patients with AIDS or AIDS-related complex, particularly in male homosexuals. It presents as purplish nodules or macules on the face, limbs, trunk or in the mouth (Fig. 3), but often also involves the internal organs and lymph notes. Kaposi's sarcoma may be due to herpes virus 8 infection. A more benign form, seen in elderly East European Jewish men, is not associated with HIV.
- *Lymphoma*: Lymphomas seen with late-phase HIV infection are often extra-nodal and sometimes cutaneous.

MANAGEMENT

Clinical diagnosis of HIV infection is confirmed by a blood test for antibod-

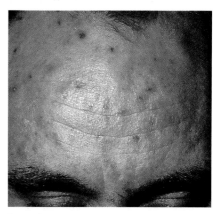

Fig. 1 **Seborrhoeic dermatitis** often seen in early and intermediate HIV infection.

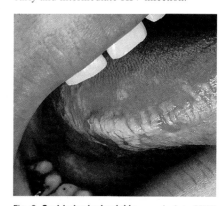

Fig. 2 **Oral hairy leukoplakia** seen in late HIV infection (AIDS).

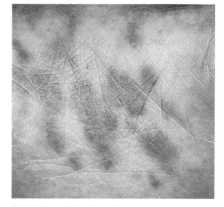

Fig. 3 **Kaposi's sarcoma** is found in intermediate and late HIV infection.

ies to the virus. Patients should be managed in departments with special experience in HIV disease. Infected individuals are counselled and sexual contacts are traced. Five years after HIV infection, 15% will have progressed to AIDS but two-thirds of the remainder will be asymptomatic. Ten years after infection, 50% will have developed AIDS, of whom 80% will have died. After AIDS has developed, mortality is high, with 50% dying in 1 year and 85% in 5 years. About 30-50% of infants born to HIV-infected women have HIV disease.

The best predictors of progression are the CD4 count (less than 250 cells/μL predicts a 66% chance of developing AIDS within 2 years) and the development of oral candidiasis.

Medical intervention is by anti-retroviral therapy (with zidovudine didanosine or zalcitabine), the prophylaxis of opportunistic infection and general support including early treatment of infections. Zidovudine (AZT) prolongs survival by 2 years. Aerosol pentamidine or oral co-tri-moxazole are effective in preventing *P. carinii* pneumonia, and ganciclovir is used to control cytomegalovirus infection. Kaposi's sarcoma may be treated with interferon alfa.

CONGENITAL IMMUNE DEFICIENCY SYNDROMES

Congenital immune deficiency syndromes are divided into:

- *B cell deficiency*: immunoglobulin deficit
- *T cell deficiency*: impairment of cell-mediated immunity, see p. 11
- *defects in effector mechanisms* such as complement or neutrophils.

Many of these conditions are very rare and present in infancy with failure to thrive. Opportunistic or pyogenic infections which often involve the skin are a feature.

Examples of these include:

- *X-linked agammaglobulinaemia*: infections occur in infancy once maternal antibodies run out.
- *IgA deficiency*: affects 1 in 700 caucasians, half get recurrent infections.
- *severe combined immuno deficiency*: fatal in infancy due to overwhelming infection unless treated by bone marrow transplant.
- *Wiskott-Aldrich syndrome*: X-linked with T-cell defects and an associated eczema.
- *chronic mucocutaneous candidiasis*: seen with severe

immune deficiencies, multiple endocrine dysfunction, or occurring sporadically: mainly due to a T-cell defect. Candidiasis usually involves the mouth, skin or nails (Fig. 4).

- *chronic granulomatous disease*: phagocytosis is defective.

SKIN SIGNS OF IMMUNOSUPPRESSION FOR ALLOGRAFTS

The use of corticosteroids, azathioprine and cyclosporin for the suppression of allograft rejection is well established. Cutaneous side-effects include not only drug eruptions and side-effects from the drugs but also infections and tumours which develop

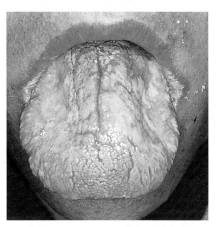

Fig. 4 **Chronic mucocutaneous candidiasis**, mainly due to a T-cell defect.

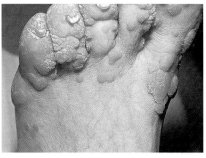

Fig. 5 **Extensive viral warts** in an immunosuppressed renal transplant patient.

due to impairment of immune surveillance, and graft-versus-host disease, which is a manifestation of an immune reaction against the host's body by the grafted tissue (p. 79). Recipients of renal allografts seem to be at particular risk for developing skin cancers. Specific skin problems in immunosuppressed allograft recipients include:

- *infections and infestations*: herpes zoster (p. 51), herpes simplex, and cytomegalovirus infection may be reactivated with immuno-suppressive therapy. Boils and cellulitis are common, and crusted 'Norwegian' scabies (p. 111) may occur.
- *human papilloma virus infection*: about 50% of renal transplant patients have viral warts (Fig. 5). These may be associated with actinic keratoses or other dysplastic lesions on sun-exposed sites. The human papilloma virus acts as a carcinogen along with sun exposure.
- *skin cancers*: the risk of skin cancer in renal transplant recipients is increased 20-fold compared with the normal population. Squamous-cell carcinomas (Fig. 6) are more common than basal-cell carcinomas. The tumours may look banal but behave aggressively.
- *graft-versus-host disease*: see p. 79.

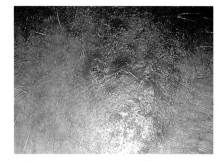

Fig. 6 **Squamous cell carcinoma** associated with immunosuppression in a renal transplant recipient.

HIV disease and immunosuppression

- *HIV infection* may be asymptomatic for several years. Skin signs of early HIV disease include dry skin and seborrhoeic dermatitis, signs of late disease are extensive infections, oral candidiasis and Kaposi's sarcoma. Treatment includes anti-retroviral therapy and the prevention of opportunistic infection.
- *Congenital immunodeficiency syndromes* are rare, often present with failure to thrive in infancy, and are associated with opportunistic or pyogenic infections.
- *Immunosuppression for allografts* is associated particularly with human papilloma virus infection, squamous-cell carcinomas or dysplastic lesions, and graft-versus-host disease.

FUNGAL INFECTIONS

Fungal infection in humans is common and mainly due to two groups of fungi:

- *dermatophytes* — multicellular filaments or hyphae
- *yeasts* — unicellular forms that replicate by budding.

These are usually confined to the stratum corneum, but deep mycoses invade other tissues (p. 57). Pityriasis versicolor, due to a yeast, is described on page 38.

DERMATOPHYTE INFECTIONS

Dermatophyte fungi reproduce by spore formation. They infect the stratum corneum, nail and hair, and induce inflammation by delayed hypersensitivity or by metabolic effects. There are three genera:

- *Microsporum* infect skin and hair
- *Trichophyton* infect skin, nail and hair
- *Epidermophyton* infect skin and nail.

Thirty species are pathogenic in humans. Zoophilic species (transmitted to humans from animals), e.g. *T. verrucosum* (Fig. 1), produce more inflammation than anthropophilic (human only) species.

Pathology

Dermatophytes inhabit keratin as branching hyphae, identifiable on microscopy. Skin scrapings, placed on a slide with 10% aqueous potassium hydroxide (to separate the keratinocytes) and a coverslip, are examined microscopically for hyphae (p. 106). The dermatophyte is identified by culturing the scrapings on medium (e.g. Sabouraud's) for 3 weeks.

Clinical presentation

Tinea (Latin: *worm*) denotes a fungal skin infection which is often annular. The exact features depend on the site. The various presentations include:

- *Tinea corporis (trunk and limbs).* Single or multiple plaques, with scaling and erythema especially at the edges, characterize this presentation. The lesions enlarge slowly, with central clearing, leaving a ring pattern, hence 'ringworm' (Figs 1 and 2). Pustules or vesicles may be seen.
- *Tinea cruris (groin).* This is more common in men and is often seen in athletes ('jock itch') who may also have tinea pedis. It spreads to the upper thigh but rarely involes the scrotum. The advancing edge may be scaly, pustular or vesicular. Causative organisms are shown in Table 1.

- *Tinea incognito.* Fungal infection can be modified in appearance and spread by the anti-inflammatory effect of a topical steroid.
- *Tinea manuum (hand).* Typically, this appears as a unilateral, diffuse powdery scaling of the palm (Fig. 3). *T. rubrum* is often the cause. Tinea pedis may co-exist.
- *Tinea capitis (scalp/hair).* See pages 63 and 107.
- *Tinea unguium (nails).* See page 64.
- *Tinea pedis (athlete's foot).* Athlete's foot (p. 106) is common in adults (especially young men), rare in children and predisposed to by communal washing, swimming baths, occlusive footwear and hot weather. Itchy interdigital maceration, usually of the 4th/5th toeweb space, is most frequent, but diffuse 'moccasin' involvement is seen. Recurrent vesicles also occur, sometime with pompholyx as an id reaction. The commonest organisms are *T. rubrum, T. mentagrophytes var. interdigitale* and *Epidermophyton floccosum.*

The differential diagnoses of superficial mycoses are shown Table 1. Microscopy and culture of skin scrapings is

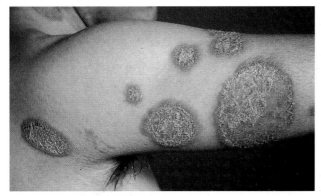

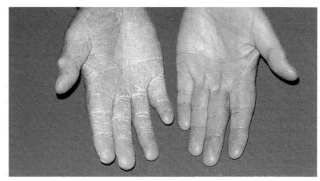

Fig. 3 **Unilateral tinea manuum caused by *T. rubrum*.**

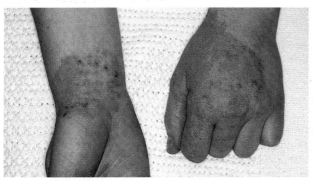

Fig. 1 **Tinea corporis.** The infection is due to animal ringworm (*T. verrucosum*) and shows intense inflammation.

Fig. 2 **Tinea corporis with a well-defined edge and some central clearing.**

Table 1 **Superficial mycoses: causative organisms and differential diagnosis**

Area	Commonest organism	Differential diagnosis
Body/limbs (corporis)	*T. verrucosum, M. canis, T. rubrum*	Discoid eczema, psoriasis, pityriasis rosea
Feet (pedis)	*T. rubrum, T. interdigitale, E. floccosum*	Contact dermatitis, psoriasis, pompholyx, erythrasma
Groin (cruris)	*T. rubrum, E. floccosum, T. interdigitale*	Intertrigo, candidiasis, erythrasma
Hand (manuum)	*T. rubrum*	Chronic eczema, psoriasis, granuloma annulare
Nail (unguium)	*T. rubrum, T. interdigitale*	Psoriasis, trauma, candidiasis
Scalp (capitis)	*M. canis, M. audouinii, T. tonsurans, T. schoenleinii*	Alopecia areata, psoriasis, seborrhoeic eczema, furunculosis

often helpful. Wood's ultraviolet light examination is used for tinea capitis, especially for screening during outbreaks. Hair infected by *M. audouinii* and *M. canis* fluoresces green, but *T. tonsurans* does not fluoresce.

Management

Humid and sweaty conditions, including occlusive footwear, should be minimized, and dusting powder may help to keep the feet or body folds dry. Minor fungal infections respond to topical treatments, but widespread involvement or diseases of the nails or scalp requires systemic therapy.

Topical therapy

Whitfield's ointment (containing benzoic acid) and Magenta paint have been replaced by the imidazoles (e.g. Canesten, Daktarin, Ecostatin and Exelderm). Tinea corporis, tinea pedis and tinea cruris respond to topical creams, sprays or powders. Terbinafine (Lamisil) cream was recently introduced (p. 106). Amorolfine (Loceryl) nail lacquer, applied once weekly, produces a 40–50% cure for tinea unguium. Before antifungal agents, scalp ringworm sometimes required X-irradiation.

Systemic therapy

Tinea capitis, tinea manuum, tinea unguium and extensive tinea corporis often require systemic treatment. Tinea corporis and tinea manuum respond to griseofulvin 500mg once a day (for an adult) for 1–2 months. Scalp ringworm requires 3 months treatment, fingernail involvement 4–8 months and toenail infection 18 months. In the elderly, fungal toenail infection often does not require any therapy. However, griseofulvin is effective in 30% of toenail infections and 70% of fingernail infections. Griseofulvin may cause headache, nausea, gastrointestinal upset and photosensitivity, and can interact with warfarin, oral contraceptives and phenobarbitone.

The new anti-fungal agents, with greater efficacy and fewer side-effects, are usually preferred to griseofulvin, except in children. Terbinafine (Lamisil) 250mg daily, and itraconazole (Sporanox) 100mg daily, may be used for tinea corporis, cruris, manuum and pedis, given for 2–4 weeks. Tinea unguium responds to terbinafine (250mg daily) or itraconazole (200mg daily) for 6–12 weeks.

Ketoconazole (Nizoral), though effective, is limited in use by hepatotoxicity.

CANDIDA ALBICANS INFECTION

Candida albicans is a ubiquitous commensal of the mouth and gastrointestinal tract which can produce opportunistic infection. Predisposing factors include:

- moist and opposing skin folds
- obesity or diabetes mellitus
- immunosuppression (p. 53)
- pregnancy
- poor hygiene
- humid environment
- wetwork occupation
- use of broad-spectrum antibiotic.

Clinical presentation

In infection, hyphal forms of *C. albicans* are seen in the stratum corneum. Infection may present as:

- *Genital.* Thrush commonly appears as an itchy, sore vulvovaginitis. White plaques adhere to inflamed mucous membranes and a white vaginal discharge may occur. Males develop similar changes on the penis. It can be spread by sexual intercourse.
- *Intertrigo.* Super-infection with *C. albicans*, and often also with bacteria, gives a moist, glazed and macerated appearance to the submammary, axillary or inguinal body folds. The interdigital clefts are involved (Fig. 4) in wetworkers who do not dry their hands properly.
- *Muco-cutaneous candidiasis.* This rare, sometimes inherited disorder of immune deficiency starts in infancy. Chronic *C. albicans* intertrigo with nail and mouth infections are seen.
- *Oral.* White plaques adhere to an erythematous buccal mucosa. Broadspectrum antibiotics, false teeth and poor oral hygiene predispose. Angular stomatitis may co-exist.
- *Paronychia.* See page 64.
- *Systemic.* Systemic candidiasis can occur in immunosuppressed patients. Red nodules are seen in the skin.

Management

Candida albicans infections must be differentiated from other conditions (Table 2). General measures are important. Body folds are separated and kept dry with dusting powder. Hands are dried carefully (p. 35) and oral hygiene improved. Systemic antibiotics may need to be stopped. Specific agents against candida are used topically and systemically.

Topical therapy

Magenta paint is useful for body folds, but is messy because of its colour. Imidazoles are effective and available as creams, powders and lotions. For oral candida, use amphotericin, nystatin or miconazole as lozenges, suspension or gels.

Systemic therapy

Bowel carriage may be reduced in recurrent candidiasis by oral nystatin. Itraconazole 100mg daily, or fluconazole (Diflucan) 50mg daily, but not griseofulvin, can be given as a short course for persistent *C. albicans* infections and in the long term for mucocutaneous candidiasis. Vaginal candidiasis is treated by a single dose of 500mg clotrimazole (Canesten) or 150mg econazole (Gyno-Pevaryl) as a pessary, or with itraconazole or fluconazole by mouth.

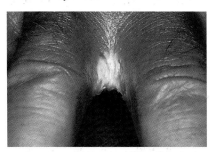

Fig. 4 **Intertrigo of the interdigital cleft due to** *C. albicans*.

Table 2 **Differential diagnosis:** *C. albicans* infections

Variant	Differential diagnosis
Genital	Psoriasis, lichen planus, lichen sclerosus
Intertrigo	Psoriasis, seborrhoeic dermatitis, bacterial secondary infection
Oral	Lichen planus, epithelial dysplasia
Paronychia	Bacterial infection, chronic eczema

Fungal infections

- Dermatophytes infect the feet, groin, body, nails, hands and scalp. The commonest dermatophyte pathogens are *T. rubrum, T. mentagrophytes var. interdigitale* and *E. floccosum*.
- Topical imidazoles and oral griseofulvin are effective for most dermatophyte infections.
- *C. albicans* produces opportunistic infection of the body folds, mouth, genitals and nail fold. These are predisposed to by humidity, obesity, diabetes and oral antibiotic therapy.
- Topical imidazoles are usually effective for candidiasis.

TROPICAL INFECTIONS AND INFESTATIONS

Infections constitute one of the biggest problems in dermatology in tropical Third World regions. Leprosy, for example, despite being a treatable disease, continues to ravage in many parts of the globe.

However, tropical infections may also be seen in countries in which they are non-endemic — amongst visitors and immigrants, or when acquired abroad by the indigenous population.

LEPROSY

Leprosy is a chronic disease caused by *Mycobacterium leprae*. This is an acid and alcohol fast bacillus which cannot be cultured in the laboratory. Infection is spread by nasal droplets and the incubation period is several years. The disease is usually acquired in childhood, as the risk to exposed adults is about 5%. Leprosy is no longer endemic in northern Europe, but it does occur in tropical and sub-tropical areas throughout the world. The manifestation of the disease depends on the degree of the delayed (type IV) hypersensitivity response in the infected individual. Those with strong cell-mediated immunity develop the tuberculoid type, whereas those in whom the cell-mediated reactivity is poor develop lepromatous leprosy. Borderline lesions are seen in those whose immune state is in-between.

M. leprae has a predilection for nerves and the dermis, but in the lepromatous type, infection may be much more widespread. Tuberculoid leprosy is characterized by a granulomatous

reaction in the nerves and dermis with no acid-fast bacilli demonstrated with the Ziehl-Neelsen stain. In contrast, bacilli are plentiful in the dermis of lepromatous type, and large numbers of macrophages are seen on microscopy.

Clinical presentation

Tuberculoid leprosy affects the nerves and the skin. Nerves may be thickened and anaesthesia or muscle atrophy are found. Skin lesions often occur on the face, and as few as one or two may be seen. They usually take the form of raised red plaques with a hypopigmented centre which typically is dry and hairless (Fig. 1). Sensation may be impaired within the plaque.

The skin lesions of *lepromatous leprosy* are multiple and take the form of macules, papules, nodules and plaques. They are symmetrical and tend to involve the face, arms, legs and buttocks. Sensation is not impaired. Untreated, the condition is infectious from the nasal involvement. Progression gives a thickened furrowed appearance to the face (leonine facies) with loss of eyebrows (Fig. 2). *Borderline leprosy* shows features intermediate between lepromatous and tuberculoid.

Leprosy must be distinguished from a variety of other dermatological conditions (Table 1).

Complications

Tuberculoid leprosy may result in bone damage of a hand or foot from repeated trauma to an insensitive

area. In lepromatous leprosy, nasal damage may progress to a saddle nose defect. Ichthyosis, testicular atrophy and leg ulcers are seen. A peripheral neuropathy leads to shortening of the toes and fingers from repeated trauma. Lepra reactions, which result from an up-grading or a down-grading of the immune response, can produce nerve destruction or acute skin lesions.

Management

Lepromatous leprosy is treated with rifampicin, dapsone and clofazimine. Treatment is for at least 2 years, continued until skin smears are negative. Tuberculoid leprosy responds to rifampicin and dapsone, given for 6–12 months. The complications of leprosy may require the skills of rehabilitation specialists and orthopaedic and plastic surgeons.

In countries where leprosy is endemic, the education of the public about the disease is important in reducing the stigma attached to sufferers. Public health programmes aimed at leprosy control are active in several countries.

LEISHMANIASIS

Leishmaniasis is a disease caused by Leishmania protozoa, which are transmitted by sand fly bites. It exists in tropical and sub-tropical areas in either a cutaneous, mucocutaneous or a visceral form. Three protozoa cause disease:

- *Leishmania tropica* causes the cutaneous 'oriental sore' and is seen around the Mediterranean coast, in the Middle East and in Asia.
- *L. braziliensis*, endemic in central and South America, leads to cutaneous and mucosal disease.
- *L. donovani* is widely distributed in

Table 1 **Differential diagnosis of leprosy**

Type of leprosy	Differential diagnosis
Tuberculoid	Vitiligo, pityriasis versicolor, pityriasis alba, sarcoidosis, lupus vulgaris, granuloma annulare, post-inflammatory hypopigmentation
Lepromatous	Disseminated cutaneous leishmaniasis, yaws, guttate psoriasis, discoid lupus erythematosus, mycosis fungoides

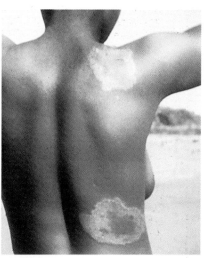

Fig. 1 **Hypopigmented plaques of tuberculoid leprosy.**

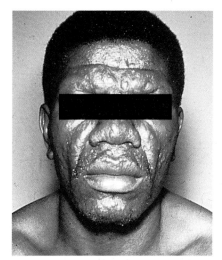

Fig. 2 **The leonine facies of lepromatous leprosy.**

Asia, Africa and South America, and causes visceral disease (kala-azar) with associated skin lesions.

Clinical presentation

Oriental sore is a common infection in endemic areas — normally affecting children, who subsequently develop immunity. In non-endemic regions, it is not infrequently seen in travellers after a Mediterranean holiday. The face, neck or arms are usually affected. At the site of inoculation, a red or brown nodule appears which either ulcerates or spreads slowly to form a crust-topped plaque (Fig. 3). Untreated, the lesion will heal in 6–12 months, although a chronic form is seen. In *mucocutaneous leishmaniasis*, the skin lesion resembles an oriental sore, but, subsequently, necrotic ulcers affect the nose, lips and palate with deformity. *Kala-azar* principally affects children and has a significant mortality. It causes hepatomegaly, splenomegaly, anaemia and debility. The cutaneous signs are patchy pigmentation on the face, hands and abdomen.

Leishmaniasis must be distinguished from some other disorders (Table 2).

Management

Cutaneous leishmaniasis may heal spontaneously, and small areas respond to cryotherapy. When specific treatment is needed, it is usual to give a pentavalent antimony compound (Pentostam) intravenously for 10–21 days. The treatment for the mucocutaneous and visceral forms is similar.

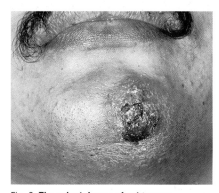

Fig. 3 **The oriental sore of cutaneous leishmaniasis.**

LARVA MIGRANS

Larva migrans is a 'creeping' eruption due to penetration of the skin by the larva stage of animal hookworms. Larva migrans is often acquired from tropical beaches where ova from the hookworms of dogs and cats have hatched into larvae which are able to penetrate the human skin. Penetration usually occurs on the feet. The larvae advance at the rate of a few millimetres a day in a serpiginous route causing red intensely itchy tracks to appear (Fig. 4). They eventually die spontaneously after a few weeks, as they cannot complete their life cycle in humans.

Topical 10% thiabendazole cream, or oral albendazole, 400 mg daily for 3 days, are usually effective.

DEEP MYCOSES

Deep mycoses are defined as the invasion of living tissue by fungi, causing systemic disease. Brief details are given in Table 3.

FILARIASIS

Filariasis is seen in the tropics and is often due to the nematode worm,

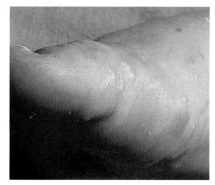

Fig. 4 **Larva migrans.** Seen in a child who had just visited beaches in the West Indies.

Wuchereria bancrofti. Lymphatic damage ultimately results in gross oedema of the legs and scrotum ('elephantiasis'). Treatment is with diethylcarbamazine.

ONCHOCERCIASIS

Onchocerciasis is a disease affecting the eyes and the skin, caused by the worm, *Onchocerca volvulus*. It is endemic in Africa and Central America and is an important cause of blindness. A gnat transmits the worm to humans. An itchy papular eruption is followed by dermal nodules with lichenification and pigmentary change. Microfilariae invade the eye and result in blindness.

Ivermectin, as a single dose, is the drug of choice for onchocerciasis. Retreatment at 6 or 12 monthly intervals may be needed until the worms die out.

Tropical infections

- *Leprosy*: tuberculoid and lepromatous forms mainly affect the skin and nerves; treatment with dapsone, rifampicin and clofazimine.
- *Leishmaniasis*: cutaneous, mucocutaneous and visceral types; treatment is with Pentostam.
- *Larva migrans*: creeping eruption due to animal hookworms; responds to thiabendazole cream or oral albendazole.
- *Deep mycoses*: serious infections which may be difficult to eradicate.
- *Onchocerciasis*: an important cause of blindness; skin shows lichenified nodules and pigmentary changes. Treatment is with ivermectin.

Table 2 **Differential diagnosis of leishmaniasis**

Variant	Differential diagnosis
Cutaneous	Lupus vulgaris, leprosy, discoid LE
Mucocutaneous	Syphilis, yaws, leprosy, blastomycosis
Kala-azar	Leprosy

Table 3 **The deep mycoses**

Mycosis	Clinical features	Management
Actinomycosis	Induration and scarring with multiple sinuses discharging yellow granules, particularly around the jaw, chest and abdomen	Long term high dose penicillin, surgical excision
Blastomycosis	Ulcerated discharging nodules which show central clearing with scarring; may spread from pulmonary infection	Systemic amphotericin B or itraconazole
Histoplasmosis	Seen in immunosuppressed patients who develop lung disease with granulomatous skin lesions	Systemic ketoconazole or itraconazole
Mycetoma	A chronic granulomatous infection usually of the foot, due to several types of fungi; nodules with sinuses, ulceration and tissue necrosis result	Depends on the fungus; surgical excision, dapsone, co-trimoxazole or rifampicin may help
Sporotrichosis	An abcess forms with nodules subsequently occurring proximally along the line of lymphatic drainage	Potassium iodide or itraconazole

INFESTATIONS

Infestation is defined as the harbouring of insect or worm parasites in or on the body. Worms — on or in the skin — are infrequent except in tropical countries. Insect life on the skin is usually transient in temperate climes, although a mite (*Demodex folliculorum*) may live harmlessly in facial hair follicles.

Insects cause a variety of skin reactions (Table 1). Contact with an insect or an insect bite can produce a chemical effect, such as a bee sting, or an irritant effect such as dermatitis from contact with a caterpillar or blistering due to cantharadin released from a crushed beetle. Contact may also cause an immune-mediated response.

Insects also act as vectors of skin disease, as in Lyme disease (p. 47), when animal ticks transmit *Borrelia burgdorferi*. They may involve the skin directly by burrowing (e.g. scabies) or by laying eggs in the skin (myiasis).

INSECT BITES

The cutaneous reaction following the bite of an insect is due to a pharmacological, irritant or allergic response to the introduced foreign material.

Clinical presentation

The lesions of insect bites vary from itchy wheals (Fig. 1) through papules

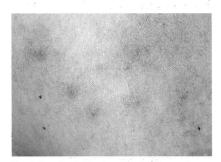

Fig. 1 **Papular urticaria, showing grouped lesions.**

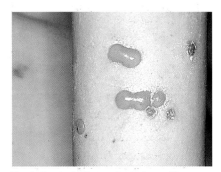

Fig. 2 **Grouped blisters due to insect bites.**

Table 1 **Insect effects on the skin**

Insect	Effect
Animal ticks	Bites, disease vector
Ants, bedbugs, fleas	Bites
Bees, wasps	Stings
Caterpillars	Dermatitis
Cheyletiella	Papular urticaria
Demodex folliculorum	Normal inhabitant
Food/harvest mites	Bites
Lice	Infestation (bites), disease vector
Mosquitoes	Bites, myiasis, disease vector
Sarcoptes scabei	Scabies

to quite large bullae (Fig. 2). The morphology will depend on the insect (Table 1) and the type of response elicited. Insect bites are usually grouped or track up a limb. Papular urticaria defines recurrent itchy urticated papules on the limbs or trunk, quite often in a child. The culprits, which may be difficult to trace, include garden insects, fleas or mites on household pets. Bedbugs cause bites on the face, neck and hands. They lie inactive in crevices in furniture during the day and emerge at night. Secondary bacterial infection of excoriated insect bites is common.

Differential diagnosis

The linear or grouped nature of the lesions is usually suggestive, but sometimes urticaria, scabies, atopic eczema or dermatitis herpetiformis may need to be considered.

Management

Elimination of the cause is often not easy, as the insects are difficult to trace. Household pets must be inspected and treated if necessary. Cat fleas exist for months on carpets without a cat being present. Birds nesting or perching by a window can introduce *Cheyletiella* into a house. An individual with insect bites can be helped by Eurax hydrocortisone cream or calamine lotion.

LICE INFESTATION (PEDICULOSIS)

Lice are flat, wingless, blood-sucking insects (Fig. 3). Their eggs (nits) are laid on hairs or clothing. There are two anthropophilic species:

- pubic louse
- body louse (the head louse is a variant).

Head lice are common amongst school children and spread by head-to-head contact. The nits are often easier to see than the lice. The body louse is mainly seen in vagrants who live in unhygienic or poor social conditions. Spread is by infested bedding or clothing. The pubic louse is sexually transmitted and is mostly found in young adults. Lice induce intense itching which, through scratching, results in excoriation and secondary infection.

Clinical presentation

The itching of head lice usually starts at the sides and back of the scalp. Scratching results in secondary infection which may cause matted hair. Body lice result in excoriations on the trunk and, in chronic infestation, lichenification and pigmentation. The lice are found in the seams of clothes. Pubic lice, known colloquially as 'crabs', result in severe pruritus with secondary eczema and infection. They may involve the eyelashes. Lice infestation should not be confused with other conditions (Table 2).

Table 2 **Differential diagnosis of pediculosis**

Louse infestation	Differential diagnosis
Body louse	Scabies, chronic eczema
Head louse	Impetigo, eczema
Pubic louse	Scabies, eczema

Management

Head lice are treated with malathion or carbaryl lotion, applied to the scalp for 12 hours, washed out and repeated in 7 days if necessary. Permethrin or

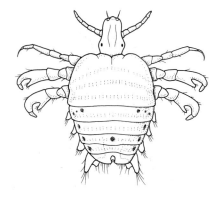

Fig. 3 **The female pubic louse.**

phenothrin are alternatives. Nits are removed with a comb. Contacts are also treated. Body lice are eradicated by treating the clothing with tumble-drying, laundering or dry-cleaning. Lindane or permethrin lotions may be used on the skin. Infestation with pubic lice requires the application of malathion, lindane or carbaryl aqueous lotions to all the body. Sexual partners should be treated.

SCABIES

The scabies mite, *Sarcoptes scabei var hominis*, is 0.4mm in length (Fig. 4) and is spread by direct physical transfer, including sexual contact. The fertilized female mite burrows through the stratum corneum at the rate of 2mm per day, laying 2 or 3 eggs each day. The eggs hatch after 3 days into larvae which form shallow pockets in the stratum corneum where they moult and mature within about 2 weeks. The mites mate in the pockets; the male dies but the fertilized female burrows and continues the cycle. After first being infested, it takes 4 to 6 weeks for the hypersensitivity reaction to the mite, and the intense itching that it causes, to develop. On average, about 12 mites are present at the itching stage but it can be many more.

Clinical presentation

The irregular, tortuous and slightly scaly burrows measure up to 1cm long. They are commonest on the sides of fingers (Fig. 5), wrists, ankles and nipples, and on the genitalia where they form rubbery nodules. Small vesicles are often seen. Itching induces excoriations (Fig. 6). In infants, the feet are frequently involved and the face can be affected. The mite is occasionally visible as a white dot at the end of a burrow. If extracted with a needle and viewed under a microscope the diagnosis is irrefutable.

Scabies is often accompanied by an ill-defined eczematous urticated papular hypersensitivity reaction on the trunk. Untreated, scabies becomes chronic.

Differential diagnosis

Other intensely itchy eruptions, such as lichen planus, dermatitis herpetiformis, papular urticaria and eczema, may need to be considered, but only scabies shows burrows. Animal scabies, due to animal mites, causes an itchy eruption, but burrows are absent.

Complications

Scabies commonly becomes secondarily infected. In institutionalized or immunosuppressed patients, very large numbers of mites proliferate to produce an extensive crusted eruption known as 'Norwegian' scabies (p. 111).

Patients commonly feel itchy for some days even after adequate treatment, and pruritic non-infested 'post-scabetic' nodules may persist for weeks. Scabicides often cause an irritant dermatitis and care must be taken to distinguish this from persistent or recurrent infestation.

Management

An adequate application technique and the treatment of all contacts are most important in the treatment

of scabies. If either is lacking, persistence or re-infestation may result. An instruction leaflet for patients is helpful. Lindane (Quellada), malathion (Prioderm) and permethrin (Lyclear) are popular. Crotamiton (Eurax), benzyl benzoate (Ascabiol) and 10% sulphur ointment are alternatives. Lindane is not recommended for pregnant women, children under 10 years, and those with a low body weight or epilepsy. The suggested technique is as follows:

- apply the lotion or cream to the entire body surface from the neck down
- treat the face and scalp in infants, the elderly and the immunosuppressed
- leave the lotion on for 24 hours and then wash off in the bath or shower
- if the hands are washed during this period, re-apply the lotion or cream
- a repeat after 1 week is sometimes suggested but usually is unnecessary if the first treatment was adequate.

Recently infested individuals do not itch, and close contacts (such as the whole family) and sexual partners need treatment. Scabies often breaks out in old peoples homes or geriatric wards and presents the problem of how far to extend the therapeutic net. The safe rule is to treat all members of a ward or home, including nurses, who have contact with the index case. Clothing and bedding is laundered. The mite dies within a few days away from the skin.

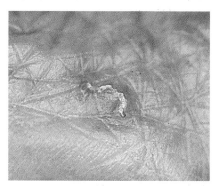
Fig. 5 **A scabetic burrow on the side of the finger of an elderly patient.**

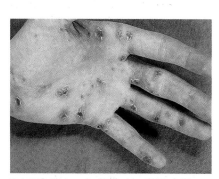
Fig. 6 **Multiple excoriations on the hand due to scabies infestation.**

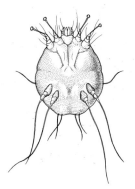
Fig. 4 **The female scabies mite.**

Infestations

- *Insect bites* present on the trunk and limbs as grouped, itchy, often blistering, papules.
- *Head lice* infestation is transmitted between school children by head contact. Secondary infection is common.
- *Body lice* occur in those living in poor social conditions and produce excoriation and lichenification.
- *Pubic lice* are sexually transmitted and present with pruritus and secondary infection.
- *Scabies* is spread by direct transfer and is intensely itchy. All contacts need treatment.

SEBACEOUS AND SWEAT GLANDS — Acne, Rosacea and Other Disorders

ACNE

Acne is a chronic inflammation of the pilosebaceous units, producing comedones, papules, pustules, cysts, and scars. It affects nearly every adolescent. Acne has an equal sex incidence and tends to affect women earlier than men, although the peak age for clinical acne is 18 years in both sexes. Acne results from:

- increased sebum excretion
- pilosebaceous duct hyperkeratosis
- colonization of the duct with *Propionibacterium acnes*
- release of inflammatory mediators (including cytokines).

In acne, the androgen-sensitive pilosebaceous unit (p. 4) shows a hyper-responsiveness that results in increased sebum excretion. Factors in sebum induce comedones, and *P. acnes* initiates inflammation through chemical mediators including enzymes (e.g. lipase) and prostaglandins (Fig. 1).

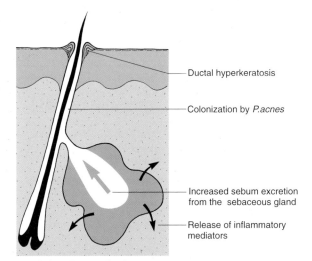

Fig. 1 **Aetiopathogenesis of acne.**

Ductal hyperkeratosis

Colonization by *P.acnes*

Increased sebum excretion from the sebaceous gland

Release of inflammatory mediators

CLINICAL PRESENTATION

Comedones are either open (black-heads: dilated pores with black plugs of melanin-containing keratin) or closed (whiteheads: small cream-coloured, dome-shaped papules). They appear at about the age of 12 years and evolve into inflammatory papules (Fig. 2), pustules or cysts (Fig. 3). The sites of predilection — the face, shoulders, back and upper chest — have many sebaceous glands. The severity of acne depends on its extent and the type of lesion, with cysts being the most destructive.

Acne usually persists until the early 20s, although in a few patients, particularly women, the disease continues into the 5th decade. Scars may follow healing, especially of cysts or abscesses. Scars may be 'ice-pick', atrophic (Fig. 4) or keloidal.

Some variants of acne are seen:

- *Acne excoriée:* due to squeezing, affects depressed or obsessional young women.
- *Chloracne:* caused by certain aromatic halogenated industrial chemicals.
- *Conglobate:* a mass of burrowing abscesses and sinuses with scarring.
- *Cosmetic:* pomade and cosmetic-induced comedonal/papular acne (mainly seen in the USA).
- *Drug-induced:* by systemic steroids, androgens and topical steroids.
- *Infantile:* mostly found on the faces of male infants. Cause: unknown.
- *Physical:* occlusion by the back of a wheel-chair or on a violinist's chin.

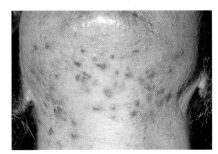

Fig. 2 **Papular-pustular acne of the chin, with some whiteheads.**

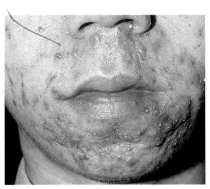

Fig. 3 **Pustulo-cystic acne on the face.**

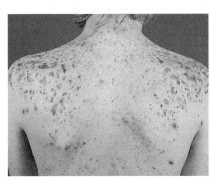

Fig. 4 **Scarring acne on the back.**

COMPLICATIONS AND DIFFERENTIAL DIAGNOSIS

Embarrassment, shame and lack of confidence are important sequelae of acne. These improve with effective treatment. The rare and severe acne fulminans, seen in adolescent males, is associated with fever, arthritis and vasculitis. Long-term antibiotic treatment may induce a Gram-negative folliculitis.

Rosacea can usually be differentiated from acne (see below). Bacterial folliculitis is more acute than acne, but the two may coexist.

MANAGEMENT

Treatment depends on the type and extent of acne and the patient's psychological state. 'Over the counter' creams have often already been used.

Local treatment is adequate for mild acne and is used with systemic drugs for more severe cases.

- *Benzoyl peroxide* (Panoxyl, Benzagel, Nericur) cream or gel, applied twice a day, works by reducing the number of *P. acnes*. It may cause irritation, contact allergy and bleach clothing.
- *Tretinoin* (Retin A cream or gel) is good at reducing the number of comedones, but may be irritant.
- *Antibiotics*, e.g. clindamycin (Dalacin T), erythromycin (Stiemycin) and tetracycline (Topicycline), can be used for mild or moderately severe acne.

● *Newer topical agents*, e.g. azelaic acid, erythromycin with zinc, isotretinoin, and nicotinamide (p.106).

Oral treatment with antibiotics, retinoids or hormones is prescribed for moderate or severe acne, acne excoriée and in depressed patients.

Antibiotics

The first-line systemic antibiotic drug is tetracycline, 500 mg twice daily (taken half an hour before food with water), given for a minimum of 4 months. Tetracyclines are contraindicated in children and in pregnancy, and may cause *C. albicans* infection or photosensitivity. Minocycline (Minocin, Aknemin, 100 mg daily) and doxycycline (Vibramycin, 50 mg once daily) are alternative tetracyclines that are better absorbed.

Erythromycin (500 mg twice daily) and trimethoprim are second-choice antibiotics. Women on oral contraceptives who take an antibiotic are advised that, if diarrhoea develops, additional contraception is needed for the rest of the menstrual cycle.

Anti-androgen

The combination of an anti-androgen and an oestrogen (cyproterone acetate, 2 mg, and ethinyl oestradiol, 35 μg: Dianette) is used in females (not males) with moderate to severe acne which is resistant to conventional therapy. The anti-androgen suppresses sebum production. Dianette is given for 6–12 months and is also a contraceptive.

Retinoid

Isotretinoin (Roaccutane) — which reduces sebum excretion, inhibits *P. acnes* and is anti-inflammatory — is a very effective treatment for acne. It is used if acne is severe or unresponsive to conventional treatment, or if acne relapses quickly once antibiotics are stopped. A course lasts 4–6 months and requires the monitoring of liver function and fasting lipids. Isotretinoin is teratogenic. Women given the drug must not be pregnant and need to take the oral contraceptive throughout treatment and for the month before and after. Common side-effects include cracked lips, dry skin, nose bleeds, hair loss and muscle aches.

Other therapies

Acne cysts may require injection with triamcinolone acetonide (a steroid), or sometimes excision or cryotherapy. Comedones can be removed using an extractor. Diet has no effect on acne.

ROSACEA

Rosacea is a chronic inflammatory facial dermatosis characterized by erythema and pustules. The cause of rosacea is unknown. Histologically, dilated dermal blood vessels, sebaceous gland hyperplasia and an inflammatory cell infiltrate are seen. Sebum excretion is normal.

CLINICAL PRESENTATION

Rosacea has an equal sex incidence. Although commonest in middle age, it also affects young adults and the elderly. The earliest symptom is flushing. Erythema, telangiectasia, papules, pustules (Fig. 5) and, occasionally, lymphoedema involve the cheeks, nose, forehead and chin. Rhinophyma-hyperplasia of the sebaceous glands and connective tissue of the nose (Fig. 5), and eye involvement by blepharitis and conjunctivitis, are complications. Sunlight and topical steroids exacerbate the condition. Rosacea persists for years, but usually responds well to treatment. Rosacea lacks the comedones of acne and occurs in an older age group. Contact dermatitis, photosensitive eruptions, seborrhoeic dermatitis and lupus erythematosus often involve the face but are more acute or scaly, or lack pustules.

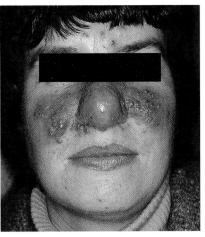

Fig. 5 **Rosacea with rhinophyma in a woman.** Rhinophyma usually affects men.

MANAGEMENT

Topically, metronidazole gel (Metrogel, Rozex) twice daily may be helpful. If this is ineffective, the usual oral treatment is tetracycline, initially 1 g daily, reducing to 250 mg daily after a few weeks and continued for 2 to 3 months. Erythromycin is an alternative. Repeated treatment is often needed. Isotretinoin can be used but is less effective than in acne. Plastic surgery is required for rhinophyma.

OTHER DISORDERS

Perioral dermatitis is characterized by papules and pustules which may occur around the mouth and chin of a woman who has used topical steroids. They will clear with oral tetracycline therapy.

Hidradenitis suppurativa is an unpleasant chronic inflammatory condition of the apocrine sweat glands of the axillae, groin and perineum. Nodules, abscesses, cysts and sinuses form and scarring results. Treatment is with topical antiseptics, systemic antibiotics and surgical excision. Conglobate acne may coexist.

Hyperhidrosis (excess sweating) due to eccrine gland overactivity is usually emotional in origin but may result from hypoglycaemia or shock. Treatment with 20% aluminium chloride in alcohol (Anhydrol Forte, Driclor) is often effective.

Sebaceous/apocrine disorders

Acne

● *Due to* pilosebaceous unit dysfunction.
● *Presentation:* comedones, pustules, cysts and scars (face, chest, trunk).
● *Treatment:* Topical treatments include benzoyl peroxide and tretinoin; Systemic treatments include antibiotics, e.g. tetracyclines or erythromycin, 'Dianette' and isotretinoin.

Rosacea

● *Affects* middle-aged or elderly.
● *Presentation:* facial erythema, telangiectasia and pustules; rhinophyma and conjunctivitis.
● *Treatment:* oral tetracycline.

Hidradenitis suppurativa

● *Presentation:* nodules or abscesses of axillae and groin.
● *Treatment:* topical antiseptics, oral antibiotics, excision.

DISORDERS OF HAIR

HAIR LOSS (ALOPECIA)

The division of alopecia into diffuse localized, and scarring or non-scarring, helps in diagnosis (Table 1).

DIFFUSE NON-SCARRING

With diffuse, non-scarring alopecia, patients usually notice excessive numbers of hairs on the pillow, brush or comb, and after washing their hair. The scalp shows a diffuse reduction in hair density. The causes are described below.

Male pattern/androgenetic alopecia

Male pattern baldness is inherited (the exact mode is unclear) and androgen-dependent. Over several cycles the androgen-sensitive follicles convert from terminal to vellus hairs. Males are affected from the second decade, and by the 7th decade, 80% have involvement. Androgenetic alopecia also occurs in females, the majority of whom are hormonally normal. It becomes more pronounced after the menopause and is present in

Table 1 **Causes of hair loss**

Type of hair loss	Causes
Diffuse non-scarring	Male pattern/androgenetic, hypothyroid, hypopituitary, hypoadrenal, drug-induced, iron deficiency, telogen and anagen effluvium, diffuse alopecia areata
Localized/non-scarring	Alopecia areata, ringworm, traumatic, hairpulling, traction, secondary syphilis
Localized/diffuse scarring	Burns, radiation, shingles, kerion, tertiary syphilis, lupus erythematosus, morphoea, pseudopelade, lichen planus

50% of 50-year-old women. In men, bitemporal recession followed by a bald crown is the usual pattern (Fig. 1); women may show this but more commonly exhibit a diffuse thinning. Most patients require no treatment, but if therapy is felt to be justified, topical minoxidil (Regaine) produces some response in a third of cases.

Endocrine and nutrition related

Endocrine disorders often present with hair loss. Underactivity of the thyroid, pituitary or adrenals can cause diffuse alopecia, as may hyperthyroidism. Androgen-secreting tumours in women produce male-pattern baldness with virilization. Malnutrition induces dry brittle hair that becomes pale or red in kwashiorkor (protein deficiency). Diffuse hair loss is also seen with iron or zinc deficiency.

Telogen effluvium

Hair follicles are not usually in phase, but, if synchronized into the telogen resting mode, they will be shed in unison about 3 months later. Such an *effluvium* results from high fever, childbirth, surgery, drugs or other stress.

Drug-induced

Abrupt cessation of growth (*anagen effluvium*) may follow ingestion of a poison such as thallium, but is more commonly drug-induced, e.g. with cytotoxics (especially cyclophosphamide), heparin, warfarin, carbimazole, colchicine and vitamin A.

LOCALIZED NON-SCARRING

Patchy hair loss is due to a variety of causes, as described below.

Alopecia areata

Alopecia areata is a common condition, associated with autoimmune disorders, in which anagen is prematurely arrested. It generally starts in the 2nd or 3rd decade and presents with sharply defined non-inflamed bald

patches on the scalp. Pathognomonic exclamation-mark hairs, which taper as they approach the scalp, are seen. The eyebrows and beard can also be affected, and nails may show pitting.

The course is unpredictable: bald patches may enlarge progressively but, for a first attack, regrowth (often initially with white hairs) is usual (Fig. 2). Pre-pubertal onset, extensive involvement (especially of the posterior scalp) and atopy signal a poor prognosis. Complete scalp alopecia (*totalis*) or loss of all bodily hair (*universalis*) are seen occasionally and, rarely, diffuse scalp alopecia occurs.

Treatment depends on the extent: if localized, spontaneous regrowth is probable and intralesional steroid (e.g. triamcinolone acetonide) may accelerate this. If extensive, therapy is less successful. PUVA or the application of sensitizers (e.g. diphencyprone) are tried, but wigs are often necessary.

Infections

Scalp ringworm infection can result in patchy hair loss, and is described below. Secondary syphilis causes a patchy alopecia.

Trauma/traction

Constantly rubbing or pulling the hair can result in its loss. Traction from tight rollers or pulling hair in a bun causes alopecia at the scalp margins.

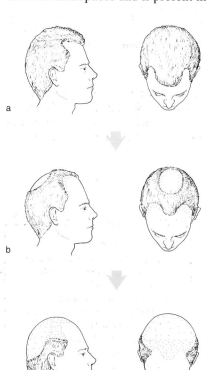

Fig. 1 **Male pattern baldness.** Hair loss may progress from bitemporal recession (**a**) to vertex involvement (**b**) to the most severe form (**c**), where only a horseshoe of hair runs from the ears to the occiput.

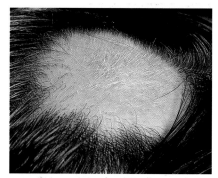

Fig. 2 **Alopecia areata showing some exclamation-mark (!) hairs and growth of white hair.**

Hair straightening, bleaching and permanent waving produce a damaged hair shaft that is easily broken.

LOCALIZED/DIFFUSE SCARRING ALOPECIA

In scarring (cicatricial) alopecia, hair follicles are destroyed. This condition can result from:

- *Burns/irradiation.* Chemical or thermal burns will scar the scalp, as may X-irradiation which, in the past, was used to induce epilation in the treatment of scalp ringworm.
- *Infection.* Shingles of the first trigeminal dermatome (p. 51), kerion (see below) and tertiary syphilis may leave a scarred scalp.
- *Lichen planus/lupus erythematosus.* Scarring alopecia, with erythema, scaling and follicular changes, is seen when these conditions affect the scalp (Fig. 3). Lesions may exist elsewhere. Topical or intralesional steroids or systemic therapies are prescribed.
- *Pseudopelade.* Pseudopelade describes a scarring alopecia which represents the end-stage of an idiopathic or unidentified destructive inflammatory process in the scalp.

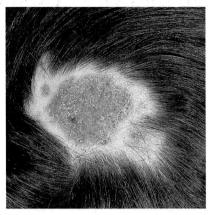

Fig. 3 **Scarring alopecia due to discoid LE, which involves the scalp with erythema and scaling.**

EXCESS HAIR (HIRSUTISM AND HYPERTRICHOSIS)

Hirsutism is the growth of terminal hair in a male pattern in a female. *Hypertrichosis* is excessive terminal hair growth in a non-androgenic distribution. Often, hirsutism is racial or idiopathic and represents an increased end-organ sensitivity to androgens (Table 2). Only a few cases are due to increased androgen secretion, although it is important to identify these. Hypertrichosis is less common and usually due to a systemic effect (Table 3).

Idiopathic hirsutism is quite common and presents with hair growth in the beard area, around the nipples and in the male pubic pattern. It frequently causes a lot of anxiety, even if mild. Virilizing features such as cliteromegaly, male-pattern baldness and a deep voice must be excluded. In hypertrichosis, fine terminal hair appears on the face, limbs and trunk (Fig. 4). Mostly it is drug-induced.

Women with a normal menstrual cycle and no signs of virilization are unlikely to have a significant endocrine cause for their hirsutism.

Table 2 **Causes of hirsutism**

Type	Example
Pituitary	Acromegaly
Adrenal	Cushing's syndrome, virilizing tumours, congenital adrenal hyperplasia
Ovarian	Polycystic ovaries, virilizing tumours
Iatrogenic	Androgens, progestogens
Idiopathic	End-organ hypersensitivity to androgens

Table 3 **Causes of hypertrichosis**

Type	Example
Localized	Melanocytic naevi, faun tail (associated with spina bifida occulta), chronic scarring or inflammation
Generalized	Malnutrition in children, anorexia nervosa, porphyria cutanea tarda, underlying malignancy, drugs, e.g. minoxidil, phenytoin, cyclosporin A

However, investigation is needed if these symptoms are present.

Treatment is often unsatisfactory. Electrolysis removes the offending hair but is time-consuming for large areas. Waxing, shaving and bleaching are other approaches. Treatment with an anti-androgen (cyproterone acetate), usually with ethinyl oestradiol, is occasionally helpful. The onset of hypertrichosis requires investigation to find the underlying cause.

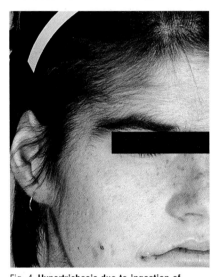

Fig. 4 **Hypertrichosis due to ingestion of minoxidil.**

OTHER DISORDERS

Hair shaft defects are rare, usually inherited, conditions of the hair shaft (e.g. monilethrix) which result in broken hairs that are brittle, beaded and look abnormal.

Dandruff is an exaggerated physiological exfoliation of fine scales from an otherwise normal scalp. More severe forms merge with seborrhoeic dermatitis of the scalp (p. 34). Psoriasis (p. 27) produces scaling and may give localized alopecia.

Tinea capitis usually affects children. Common causative organisms and recommended treatments are shown on page 55. Anthropophilic species cause defined scaly areas with slight inflammation and alopecia with broken hair shafts. Zoophilic infection with *T. verrucosum* produces an inflamed boggy, pustular swelling known as a kerion (p. 107). Scarring may result. Infection with *T. schoenleinii* causes favus — a chronic crusted scarring alopecia.

Common hair disorders

- *Male pattern baldness:* the commonest cause of hair loss; if treatment is required, topical minoxidil may help.
- *Alopecia areata:* common; discrete bald patches may show exclamation-mark (!) hairs.
- *Scarring alopecia:* needs investigation to establish the underlying cause.
- *Hirsutism:* often 'idiopathic' but investigation for androgen secretion is indicated if there are irregular menstrual periods or signs of virilism.

DISORDERS OF NAILS

CONGENITAL DISEASE

A number of usually rare congenital conditions can affect the nails. In the *nail-patella syndrome*, the nails (and patellae) are absent or rudimentary. The nails in *pachyonychia congenita* are thickened and discoloured from birth. Nail dystrophy is a feature of *dystrophic epidermolysis bullosa* (p. 87). *Racket nails*, characterized by a broad short thumb nail, is the commonest congenital nail defect. It is dominantly inherited and more common in women.

TRAUMA

Trauma, especially from sport, commonly causes nail abnormalities. *Subungual haematomas* usually occur when a fingernail has been trapped or a toenail stood on or stubbed, but the possibility of a subungual malignant melanoma must always be considered. *Splinter haemorrhages* are induced by trauma, although they also occur with infective endocarditis. Ill-fitting shoes contribute to *ingrowing toenails*, and chronic trauma predisposes to *onychogryphosis* — in which the big toenails become thickened and grow like a horn. Trauma may also induce onycholysis (separation of the nail from the nail bed). Constant picking of the thumb nail will produce *a habit-tic dystrophy* with transverse ridges and grooves. *Brittle nails* is a common complaint, usually due to repeated exposure to detergents and water, although iron deficiency, hypothyroidism and digital ischaemia are other causes.

DERMATOSES

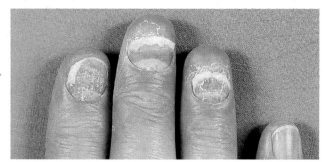

Fig. 1 **Psoriasis of the nails.** Pitting, onycholysis and brownish discoloration are apparent.

Table 1 **Nail involvement in common dermatoses**

Dermatosis	Nail changes
Alopecia areata	Fine pitting, roughness of nail surface
Darier's disease	Longitudinal ridges, triangular nicks at distal nail edge
Eczema	Coarse pitting, transverse ridging, dystrophy, shiny nails due to rubbing
Lichen planus	Thinned nail plate, longitudinal grooves, adhesion between distal nail fold and nail bed (pterygium), complete nail loss
Psoriasis	Pitting, nail thickening, onycholysis (separation of nail from nail bed), brown discoloration, subungual hyperkeratosis

The nails are commonly involved in skin disease (Figs 1 and 2), and are routinely assessed in a dermatological examination. Details are given in Table 1, and a differential diagnosis of the changes is shown in Table 2. Treatment is aimed at the associated dermatosis; care of the hands (p. 35) is especially important.

INFECTIONS

Bacterial or fungal infection may involve the nail fold (paronychia) or the nail itself.

Onychomycosis (tinea unguium)

Fungal infection of the nails (onychomycosis) increases with age — children are seldom affected. Toenails, especially the big toenails (Fig. 3), are involved more than fingernails. The process usually begins at the distal nail edge and extends proximally to involve the whole nail. The nail separates from the nail bed (onycholysis), the nail plate becomes thickened crumbly and yellow, and subungual

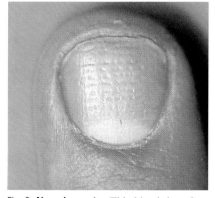

Fig. 2 **Alopecia areata.** Thimble pitting of the nail is seen.

hyperkeratosis occurs. Several — but almost never all — the toenails may be involved. Tinea pedis often co-exists, and if the fingernails are diseased, *T. rubrum* infection of the hand is usually seen. Treatment is with oral terbinafine (Lamisil) or itraconazole (Sporanox).

Chronic paronychia

Chronic paronychia of the fingernails due to *C. albicans* is often seen in wetworkers. The cuticle is lost, the prox-

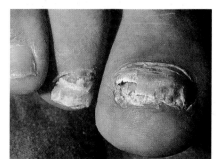

Fig. 3 **Fungal infection of toenails.** The nails are thickened, crumbly and discoloured. An adjacent nail is not affected. Dermatophytes, *C. albicans*, and, occasionally, moulds such as *Fusarium* or *Scopulariopsis brevicaulis* are causative.

imal nail fold becomes boggy and swollen (Fig. 4), and light pressure may extrude pus. The nail plate becomes irregular and discoloured. Gram-negative bacteria may be copathogens and turn the nail a blue-green colour. Management is directed towards keeping the hands dry, applying an imidazole lotion or cream twice daily to the nail fold, or oral itraconazole for 14 days (p. 106).

Table 2 **Differential diagnosis of nail changes in dermatoses and systemic disease**

Change	Description of nail	Differential diagnosis
Beau's lines	Transverse grooves	Any severe systemic illness which affects growth of the nail matrix
Brittle nails	Nails break easily, usually at distal margin	Effect of water and detergent, iron deficiency, hypothyroidism, digital ischaemia
Colour change	Black transverse bands Blue Blue-green Brown Brown 'oil-stain' patches Brown longitudinal streak Red streaks ('splinter haemorrhages') White spots White transverse bands White/brown 'half and half' nails White (leuconychia) Yellow Yellow nail syndrome (Fig. 5)	Cytotoxic drugs Cyanosis, antimalarials, haematoma Pseudomonas infection Fungal infection, stain from cigarette smoke, chlorpromazine, gold, Addison's disease Psoriasis Melanocytic naevus, malignant melanoma, Addison's disease, racial variant Infective endocarditis, trauma Trauma to nail matrix (not calcium deficiency) Heavy metal poisoning Chronic renal failure Hypoalbuminaemia (e.g. associated with cirrhosis) Psoriasis, fungal infection, jaundice, tetracycline Defective lymphatic drainage — pleural effusions may occur
Clubbing	Loss of angle between nail fold and nail plate, bulbous finger-tip, nail matrix feels spongy	*Respiratory:* bronchial carcinoma, chronic infection, fibrosing alveolitis, asbestosis; *cardiac:* infective endocarditis, congenital cyanotic defects; *other:* inflammatory bowel disease, thyrotoxicosis, biliary cirrhosis, congenital
Koilonychia	Spoon-shaped depression of nail plate	Iron deficiency anaemia; also — lichen planus and repeated exposure to detergents
Nail fold telangiectasia	Dilated capillaries and erythema at nail fold	Connective tissue disorders including systemic sclerosis, systemic LE, dermatomyositis
Onycholysis	Separation of nail from nail bed	Psoriasis, fungal infection, trauma, thyrotoxicosis, tetracyclines
Pitting	Fine or coarse pits may be seen in nail bed	Psoriasis, eczema, alopecia, lichen planus
Ridging	Transverse (across nail) Longitudinal (up/down)	Beau's lines (q.v.), eczema, psoriasis, tic-dystrophy, chronic paronychia Lichen planus, Darier's disease

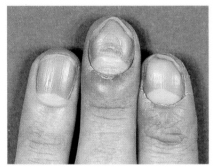

Fig. 4 *C. albicans* **is the commonest pathogen in chronic paronychia.** The nail fold is inflamed and swollen, and the nail is ridged transversely.

Acute paronychia

Acute paronychia is usually bacterial, and staphylococci are often the cause. Oral flucloxacillin or erythromycin is required.

SYSTEMIC DISEASE

Nail changes not infrequently indicate an underlying internal medical disorder. Table 2 shows some systemic associations.

TUMOURS

Tumours of the nail and nail bed are rare, but it is not uncommon to see benign tumours around the nail fold. Examples of both include:

- *Viral warts.* Periungual warts are common. Treatment is similar to that for warts elsewhere (p. 49).
- *Periungual fibromas.* These are seen in patients with tuberous sclerosis (p. 88) and appear at or after puberty.

- *Myxoid (mucous) cysts.* The cysts appear adjacent to the proximal nail fold usually on the fingers. They are fluctuant, semi-translucent papules that contain a clear gel and may arise from folds of synovium. Treatment is by cryotherapy, injection with triamcinolone acetonide (a steroid) or excision.
- *Malignant melanoma.* A subungual malignant melanoma should be excluded by biopsy if a pigmented longitudinal streak suddenly appears in a nail. An acral malignant melanoma may be amelanotic and can resemble a pyogenic granuloma or even chronic paronychia. Any atypical or ulcerating lesion around the nail fold requires a biopsy to exclude a malignant melanoma.

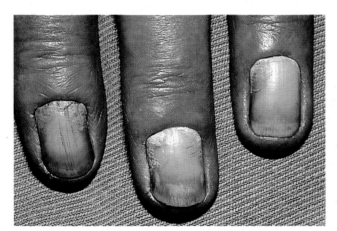

Fig. 5 **Yellow nail syndrome.** The nails grow very slowly, lymphatic drainage is abnormal and pleural effusions may occur.

Disorders of nails

- *Congenital nail problems* are uncommon except for racket nails.
- *Sports trauma* often results in subungual haematoma, onychogryphosis or onycholysis.
- *Common dermatoses* e.g. psoriasis, lichen planus and eczema, have distinctive nail changes.
- *Fungal infection* of the big toenails is common, especially in the elderly.
- *Systemic diseases* may cause nail changes which help in diagnosis.
- *Malignant melanoma* of the nail bed must be considered with any subungual pigmentation or nail destruction.

VASCULAR AND LYMPHATIC DISEASES

BLOOD VESSEL DISORDERS

ERYTHEMA

Erythema is redness of the skin, usually due to vasodilation. It may be localized, e.g. with pregnancy or liver disease (on palms), fixed drug eruption and infection (e.g. Lyme disease); or generalized, as with drug eruption, toxic erythema (e.g. viral exanthem) and connective tissue disease.

FLUSHING

Flushing is erythema due to vasodilation. The causes are:

- emotion (physiological)
- menopause (hormonal)
- foods (e.g. spices, alcohol)
- drugs (chlorpropamide, nifedipine)
- rosacea (mechanism unknown)
- carcinoid syndrome (serotonin)
- phaeochromocytoma (catecholamine).

Flushing is common and affects the face, neck and upper trunk. It is usually benign. A sudden onset and systemic symptoms (e.g. diarrhoea or fainting) mean that carcinoid syndrome or phaeochromocytoma must be excluded. In treatment, first remove the cause, e.g. spices or alcohol. Embarrassing physiological flushing may improve with a small dose of propranolol.

TELANGIECTASIA

Telangiectasia is a visible dilatation of dermal venules or, in spider naevi (Fig. 1), an arteriole. It results from:

- *congenital* (e.g. hereditary haemorrhagic telangiectasia)
- *skin atrophy* (topical steroids, ageing skin, radiation dermatitis)

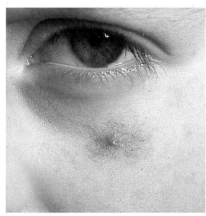

Fig. 1 **A spider naevus on the cheek of a child.**

- *excess oestrogen* (e.g. liver disease, pregnancy, 'the pill')
- *connective tissue disease* (systemic sclerosis, LE, dermatomyositis)
- *rosacea* (on the face)
- *venous disease* (lower leg).

Isolated spider naevi are common and of little significance, but their number may increase with pregnancy and liver disease. A venous lake — acquired venous ectasia — is often seen on the lower lip of the elderly. Telangiectasia is treated by fine needle cautery, hyfrecation, or laser (p. 107).

PURPURA

Purpura is a blue-brown discoloration of the skin due to the extravasation of erythrocytes (Fig. 2). It results from a variety of mechanisms:

- *Vessel wall defects*
  — vasculitis e.g. due to immune complexes
  — paraproteinaemia (e.g. cryoglobulinaemia)
  — infection (e.g. meningococcaemia)
  — raised vascular pressure (e.g. venous disease)
- *Defective dermal support*

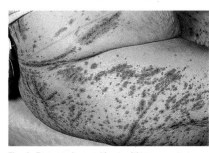

Fig. 2 **Purpura in a patient with thrombocytopenia.**

  — dermal atrophy (ageing, steroids, disease, e.g. lichen sclerosus)
  — scurvy (vitamin C deficiency)
- *Clotting defects*
  — coagulation factor deficiency (e.g. disseminated intravascular coagulation)
  — anticoagulant (heparin, warfarin)
  — thrombocytopenia of any cause
  — abnormal platelet function
- *Idiopathic pigmented purpuras.*

Petechiae are small dot-like purpura, whereas ecchymoses are more extensive. Purpura is often seen in the elderly or those on steroids, and develops spontaneously or after minor trauma. Idiopathic pigmented purpura is seen as brownish punctate lesions (capillaritis) on the legs.

Mostly there is no specific therapy. Haematological problems are treated as necessary.

RAYNAUD'S PHENOMENON

Raynaud's phenomenon is characterized by a paroxysmal vasoconstriction of the digital arteries, usually provoked by cold, in which the fingers turn white (due to ischaemia), cyanotic blue (due to capillary dilatation with a stagnant blood flow) and then red (due to reactive hyperaemia). When no cause is found, it is known as 'Raynaud's disease'. Causes include:

- *arterial occlusion:* atherosclerosis, Buerger's disease
- *connective tissue disease:* systemic sclerosis (including CREST syndrome), systemic LE (p. 76)
- *hyperviscosity syndrome:* polycythaemia, cryoglobulinaemia
- *neurological defects:* syringomyelia, peripheral neuropathy

Table 1 **Classification of blood vessel and lymphatic disorders**

Vessel	Process	Resulting lesion
Small blood vessels	Dilatation (and/or increased flow)	Erythema, flushing, telangiectasia
	Release of extracellular fluid	Urticaria (p. 72), oedema
	Release of blood	Purpura, capillaritis
	Reduced flow	Livedo reticularis, chilblains, Raynaud's phenomenon
	Inflammation damage	Vasculitis, erythema ab igne
Arteries	Atherosclerosis, Buerger's disease	Ischaemia and ulceration
	Inflammation	Vasculitis (p. 78)
Veins	Inflammation, flow reduction, clotting abnormalities	Thrombosis, skin changes, ulceration (p. 68)
	Dilatation	Venous lake
Lymphatics	Congenital hypoplasia	Lymphoedema (primary)
	Blockage/inflammation	Lymphoedema (secondary)
	Infection	Lymphangitis

- *reflux vasoconstriction:* with use of vibration tools (p. 116)
- *toxins/drugs:* ergot, vinyl chloride, beta-blockers.

Raynaud's phenomenon mostly affects women. It may be the forerunner of a connective tissue disease. The hands should be kept warm and protected from the cold. Calcium channel blockers such as nifedipine or diltiazem may help. In resistant cases, prostacyclin infusions are given.

LIVEDO RETICULARIS

Livedo reticularis is a marbled-patterned cyanosis of the skin, due to reduced arteriole blood flow. The condition has the following causes:

- *physiological* (i.e. cold-induced)
- *vasculitis* due to connective tissue disease, e.g. systemic LE and polyarteritis nodosa
- *hyperviscosity* due to cryoglobulinaemia, polycythaemia
- *Sneddon's syndrome* (livedo vasculitis with cerebrovascular disease and circulating antibodies to cardiolipin).

Cold-induced livedo reticularis gives a mottled mesh-work pattern on the outer thighs of children and is

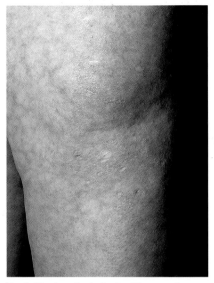

Fig. 3 **Livedo reticularis.** In this case, the condition was associated with systemic LE.

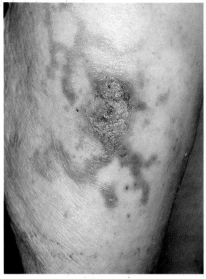

Fig. 4 **Erythema ab igne on the upper outer shin.**

reversible. Fixed livedo (Fig. 3) is due to vasculitis and requires investigation. Treatment is aimed at the underlying disease.

ERYTHEMA AB IGNE

Erythema ab igne is a reticulate pigmented erythema (Fig. 4) due to heat-induced damage. It is common on the upper outer shin of elderly folk who sit before an open fire.

CHILBLAINS

Chilblains are inflamed and painful purple-pink swellings on the fingers, toes or ears, that appear in response to cold. Chilblains result from an over-compensatory cold-induced vaso-constriction of cutaneous arterioles and venules. They occur in the winter and usually affect women. Warm housing and clothing are advised. Oral nifedipine may help.

LYMPHATIC DISORDERS

LYMPHOEDEMA

Lymphoedema is oedema, often of a limb, due to inadequate lymphatic drainage. The condition may be primary or secondary. Primary lymphoedema is the result of a congenital developmental defect. Secondary causes include:

- *recurrent infection* — lymphangitis
- *blockage* — filariasis, tumour
- *destruction* — surgery, radiation.

Primary lymphoedema presents in adolescence and may follow infection. The lower leg is commonly affected. In chronic lymphoedema, the oedema is non-pitting and fibrotic, and the overlying epidermis hyperkeratotic (Fig. 5). Lymphangiography shows the defect.

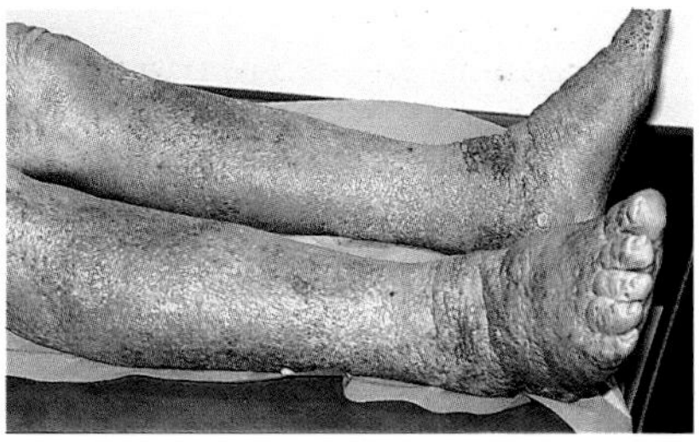

A lymphoedematous limb is at risk of repeated infection (particularly erysipelas), and long-term prophylaxis with oral penicillin V is recommended. Compression support can help. Surgical reconstruction is rarely possible.

Fig. 5 **Chronic lymphoedema of the legs, with epidermal hyperkeratosis.**

LYMPHANGITIS

Lymphangitis is defined as infection of the lymphatic vessels, usually due to streptococci. It presents as a tender red line extending proximally up a limb, usually from a focus of infection. Therapy is with intravenous antibiotic (e.g. benzylpenicillin).

Vascular and lymphatic diseases

- *Erythema:* localized, e.g. liver palms; or generalized, e.g. toxic erythema.
- *Flushing:* usually emotional; rarely carcinoid syndrome or phaeochromocytoma.
- *Telangiectasia:* commonly seen with skin atrophy, but lesions can occur with oestrogen excess or connective tissue disease.
- *Purpura:* caused by defects of the vessel wall, supporting dermis or clotting mechanism, or 'idiopathic'.
- *Livedo reticularis:* physiological or due to underlying hyperviscosity or connective tissue disorder.
- *Chilblains:* cold-induced perniosis of the fingers, toes and ears.
- *Raynaud's phenomenon:* vasoconstriction of the digital arteries with colour changes.
- *Lymphoedema:* long-term prophylaxis with antibiotics prevents recurrent infection in chronic cases.

LEG ULCERS

Leg ulcers affect 1% of the adult population and account for 1% of dermatology referrals. They are twice as common in women as in men and are a major burden on the health service. One half are venous, a tenth arterial and a quarter 'mixed' — due to venous *and* arterial disease. The remainder are due to rare causes.

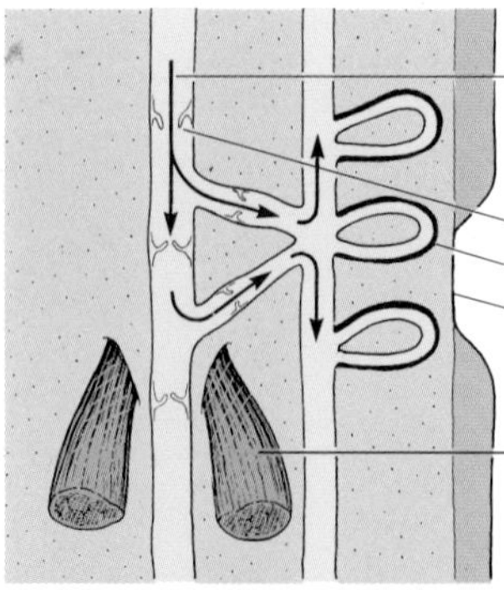

VENOUS DISEASE

Damage to the venous system of the leg results in pigment change, eczema, oedema, fibrosis and ulceration.

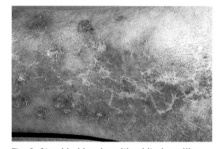

Retrograde blood flow in a deep vein

Incompetent valves
Pericapillary fibrin deposition
Ulceration

Poor muscle pump activity

Fig. 1 **The aetiopathogenesis of venous ulceration.**

AETIOPATHOGENESIS

The superficial low pressure venous system of the leg is connected to the deep higher pressure veins by perforating veins. Blood flow relies on the pumping action of surrounding muscles and the integrity of valves. Valve incompetence, occasionally congenital but usually due to damage by thrombosis or infection, results in a rise in capillary hydrostatic pressure and permeability (Fig. 1). Fibrin is deposited as a pericapillary cuff, interfering with diffusion of nutrients, and resulting in disease.

CLINICAL PRESENTATION

Venous disease usually starts in middle age and continues to later life. It is commoner in women and is predisposed to by obesity and venous thrombosis. Varicose veins are often present, but are not essential. The syndrome progresses through stages:

- *Heaviness and oedema:* early symptoms. The legs feel heavy and swell.
- *Discoloration:* brown haemosiderin deposits from extravasated red cells. Telangiectasia and white lacy scars (atrophie blanche) occur at the ankle (Fig. 2).
- *Eczema:* commonly occurs (p. 34), often complicated by allergic or irritant contact dermatitis.
- *Lipodermatosclerosis:* fibrosis of the dermis and subcutis around the ankle results in firm induration.
- *Ulceration:* often follows minor trauma, and typically affects the medial and — to a lesser extent — the lateral malleolus (Fig. 3). Neglected ulcers enlarge and may encircle the lower leg. Initially, venous ulcers are exudative, but, under favourable conditions, they

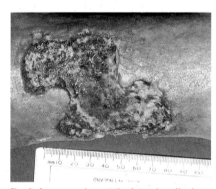

Fig. 2 **Atrophie blanche with white lace-like scarring and haemosiderin deposition.**

Fig. 3 **A venous ulcer at the lateral malleolus.**

granulate and enter a healing phase whereby the epidermis grows in from the sides and from small epithelial islands in the middle. Healing is invariably slow, often taking months. Some large ulcers never heal.
- *Post-ulcer leg:* fibrosis may lead to a slender sclerosed ankle.

DIFFERENTIAL DIAGNOSIS AND COMPLICATIONS

Venous ulcers can be differentiated from other ulcers (Table 1) by history, position and additional signs. Arterial ulcers are deep, painful and gangrenous, and situated on the foot or midshin. Complications of venous ulcers are common and include:

Table 1 **Causes of leg ulceration**

Division	Condition
Venous disease	Damaged valves (e.g. DVT), clotting disorder, congenital valve incompetence
Arterial disease	Atherosclerosis, Buerger's disease, polyarteritis nodosa
Small vessel disease	Diabetes mellitus, rheumatoid arthritis, vasculitis, sickle cell disease, hypertension
Infection	Tuberculosis, Buruli ulcer, (p. 47), mycetoma (p. 57), syphilis (p. 112)
Neuropathy	Diabetes mellitus, leprosy, syphilis (p. 112), syringomyelia
Neoplasia	Squamous cell carcinoma, Kaposi's sarcoma, malignant melanoma
Trauma	Direct injury, artefact
Unknown	Pyoderma gangrenosum (p. 85), necrobiosis lipoidica (p. 80)

- *Infections.* Ulcers are invariable colonized by bacteria. Systemic antibiotics are only needed for overt infection as suggested by a purulent discharge, a rapidly advancing ulcer edge, cellulitis or septicaemia.
- *Lymphoedema.* Lymphatic drainage is impaired in legs with chronic venous ulcers, adding to the oedema.
- *Contact dermatitis.* Contact sensitivity to topical medicaments and bandages frequently develops, especially to lanolin, neomycin and preservatives. Allergic contact dermatitis can resemble an exacerbation of venous eczema and is suspected if there is generalized secondary spread. Some local therapies, and the ulcer exudate itself, are irritant.
- *Malignant change.* Rarely, squamous cell carcinoma develops in an ulcer.

Table 2 **Topical therapy for venous ulcers**

Type of dressing or agent	Indications for use	Examples of preparations	Details of application
Antiseptic solutions	Exudative, infected or necrotic ulcers and for cleaning	0.5% silver nitrate, 0.5% acetic acid, 3% hydrogen peroxide (all aqueous)	Applied on gauze, as a wet dressing, once or twice a day, or used to irrigate the ulcer
Antiseptic and desloughing agents	Infected, sloughy or necrotic ulcers	Silver sulphadiazine (Flamazine), hydrogen peroxide (Hioxyl), proteolytic enzymes (Varidase)	Applied on a non-absorbent dressing once every 1 to 3 days
Impregnated tulle dressing	Granulating/epithelializing ulcers	Chlorhexidine (Bactigras), framycetin (Sofra-Tulle)	Applied once every 1 to 7 days
Bead preparations	Exudative, sloughy and infected ulcers	Cadexomer iodine (Iodosorb), dextranomer (Debrisan-paste)	Usually once every 1 to 7 days
Colloid or gel dressings	Granulating, sloughy and exudative ulcers	Hydrocolloid (Granuflex, Comfeel), hydrogel (Intrasite), alginate (Sorbsan, Kaltostat)	Usually once or twice a week; Granuflex/Comfeel are self-adhesive
Medicated bandages	Most ulcers, especially with eczema	Ichthammol (e.g. Ichthopaste), zinc paste (e.g. Zincaband), zinc and calamine (Calaband)	Applied in strips from foot to knee once or twice a week, often over an ulcer dressing
Low-adherent dressings	Epithelializing ulcers	Telfa, N-A Dressing, Allevyn (foam)	Once every 1 to 7 days

MANAGEMENT

Treatment of a leg ulcer is long-term and progress usually slow. The initial examination includes palpation of peripheral pulses and an assessment of contributing factors such as obesity, anaemia, cardiac failure and arthritis. Doppler studies, to exclude co-existing arterial disease, are essential when compression bandaging is proposed. Treatments are as follows:

- *Compression bandages.* These reduce oedema and promote venous return. Bandages are applied from the toes to the knee. Self-adhesive bandages (e.g. Secureforte) are preferred, and are left on for 2–7 days. A four-layer bandage technique uses a layer of orthopaedic wool (Velband), a standard crepe, an Elset elasticated bandage and an elasticated cohesive bandage (e.g. Secureforte). Arterial disease precludes compression bandaging. Once an ulcer has healed, a toe to knee compression stocking maintains venous return.
- *Elevation, exercise and diet.* Some doctors recommend rest with leg elevation. Walking is encouraged, as is dieting for obese individuals, and ankle exercises to maintain joint mobility.
- *Topical therapy.* Table 2 shows what to use and when. Venous eczema is treated with a mild/moderate potency steroid or an emollient.
- *Oral therapy.* Adequate analgesia is vital. Diuretics are given for cardiac oedema, and antibiotics for overt infection. An anabolic steroid, stanozolol (Stromba) may help lipodermatosclerosis, but side-effects (fluid retention, jaundice) limit its use. Oxerutins (Paroven) reduce capillary permeability, relieving oedema.

- *Surgery.* Vein surgery may prevent problems in younger patients, but is rarely applicable in the elderly. Split skin grafts or pinch grafts (from the thigh) are of limited use. However, experimental culturing of keratinocytes in a 'skin equivalent', to use as a graft, is promising and gives rapid pain relief.

ARTERIAL DISEASE

Lower leg ischaemia and ulceration can result from arterial disease. Ischaemia presents with claudication, coldness of the foot, loss of hair, toenail dystrophy and dusky cyanosis. Deep, sharply-defined ulcers occur on the foot or mid-shin (Fig. 4). Pulses in the legs are absent or reduced. Buerger's disease, seen in young male smokers, is a severe form of arterial disease.

Doppler studies and contrast angiography define the arterial lesions which may be amenable to vascular reconstruction or angioplasty. Compression bandaging is contraindicated.

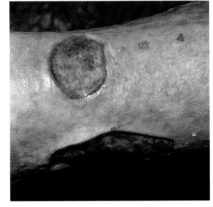

Fig. 4 **Deep arterial ulcers on the shin.**

OTHER CAUSES OF LEG ULCERATION

Vasculitic ulcers start as purpura, but become necrotic and punched out (Table 1). *Neuropathic ulcers* occur on the feet (Fig. 5) and are due to neurological disease. *Buruli ulcer* and deep mycoses are important in the tropics.

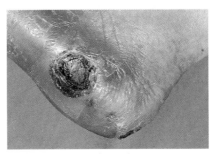

Fig. 5 **A necrotic neuropathic ulcer on the side of the foot.**

Leg ulcers

Venous ulcers
- Result from venous hypertension.
- Have associated discoloration, eczema and fibrosis.
- Occur at the medial or lateral malleolus.
- Require compression bandaging after checking Doppler pressures.
- May co-exist with arterial disease.
- May be complicated by contact allergy.

Arterial ulcers
- Are associated with other symptoms and signs of leg ischaemia.
- Occur on the foot or mid-shin.
- Are usually deep and painful.
- Prohibit compression bandaging.

PIGMENTATION

Skin colour is due to a mixture of the pigments melanin (p. 8), oxyhaemoglobin (in blood) and carotene (in the stratum corneum and subcutaneous fat). Pigmentary diseases are common and particularly distressing to those with darker skin. Disorders of pigmentation mainly involve melanocytes, but other causes are mentioned where relevant.

HYPOPIGMENTATION

Pigment loss may be generalized or patchy. Generalized hypopigmentation occurs with albinism, phenylketonuria and hypopituitarism; patchy loss is seen in vitiligo, after inflammation, following exposure to some chemicals, and with certain infections (Table 1).

VITILIGO

Vitiligo is an acquired idiopathic disorder showing white non-scaly macules. An autoimmune aetiology is suggested by the association with pernicious anaemia, thyroid disease and Addison's disease. About 30% of patients give a family history of the disorder. Melanocytes are absent from lesions on histology.

Table 1 **Causes of hypopigmentation**

Cause	Example
Chemical	Substituted phenols, hydroquinone
Endocrine	Hypopituitarism
Genetic	Albinism, phenylketonuria, tuberous sclerosis, piebaldism
Infection	Leprosy, yaws, pityriasis versicolor
Post-inflammatory	Cryotherapy, eczema, psoriasis, morphoea, pityriasis alba
Other	Vitiligo, lichen sclerosus, halo naevus

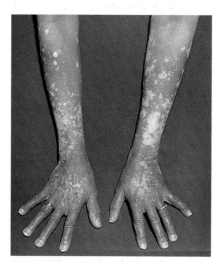

Fig. 1 **Vitiligo.** In this case there is symmetrical involvement of the forearms in a patient with a pigmented skin.

Clinical presentation

Vitiligo affects 1% of the population, is seen in all races, and is most troublesome in those with a dark skin. The sex incidence is equal and the onset, usually between 10 and 30 years of age, may be precipitated by injury or sunburn. The sharply defined white macules are often symmetrical (Fig. 1). The hands, wrists, knees, neck and areas around orifices (e.g. the mouth) are frequently affected. Occasionally, vitiligo is segmental (e.g. down an arm), generalized or universal. The course is unpredictable; areas may remain static, spread or (infrequently) repigment. In light-skinned individuals, vitiligo may only be discernible in summer, when the vitiliginous areas become sunburnt.

Differential diagnosis

Post-inflammatory hypopigmentation is often accompanied by other skin changes (Table 1). In chemical leukoderma, a history of exposure to phenolic chemicals should be sought. The hypopigmented macules of leprosy normally are anaesthetic.

Management

Treatment is unsatisfactory. Camouflage cosmetics require patience and skill to apply. Sunscreens help the lightly pigmented patient by reducing the tanning and contrast of the non-vitiligo areas. In patients with a darker skin, potent topical steroids occasionally induce re-pigmentation. PUVA, or the use of oral psoralens and natural UV radiation, sometimes helps, although it may take months. Rarely, depigmentation using monobenzyl ether of hydroquinone is considered when vitiligo is near universal and other treatments have failed.

ALBINISM

Albinism is an autosomal recessive condition in which the melanocytes fail to synthesize pigment in the epidermis, hair bulb and eye.

There are several syndromes of albinism. All are autosomal recessive and show a lack of pigment in the skin,

hair, iris and retina. Melanocyte numbers are normal, but melanosome production fails due to defective gene control of tyrosinase (p. 8).

Albinism is uncommon (the prevalence is 1/20 000), although the diagnosis is straightforward. The skin is white or pink, the hair white, and pigmentation is lacking in the eye (Fig. 2). Albinos have poor sight, photo-phobia and nystagmus. 'Tyrosinase-positive' albinos may pigment slightly with age, so that African skin becomes yellow and freckled. In the tropics, albinos risk premature skin photo-ageing and the early onset of skin tumours, especially squamous cell carcinomas.

Strict sun avoidance is essential. Opaque clothing, a wide-brimmed hat and sunscreens are needed. Prenatal diagnosis is possible.

PHENYLKETONURIA

Phenylketonuria is an autosomal recessive inborn error of metabolism. Phenylalanine hydroxylase, which converts phenylalanine into tyrosine, is deficient. Phenylalanine and metabolites accumulate and damage the developing neonatal brain. The prevalence is 1/10 000 births.

Phenylketonuria is detected after birth by routine screening tests. Untreated, mental retardation and choreoathetosis develop. Patients have fair hair and skin, due to impaired melanin synthesis. Atopic eczema is common. A low phenylalanine diet, given early, prevents neurological damage.

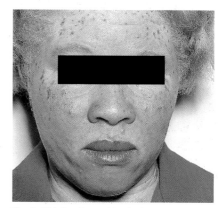

Fig. 2 **Albinism in an Afro-Caribbean patient.**

HYPERPIGMENTATION

Hyperpigmentation is mostly hypermelanosis (Table 2), but sometimes other pigments colour the skin, e.g. iron deposition (with melanin) in haemochromatosis, and carotene (causing an orange discoloration) in carotenaemia — usually due to eating too many carrots.

FRECKLES AND LENTIGINES

Freckles are small, light-brown macules, typically facial, which darken on sun exposure. Lentigines are also brown macules but are scattered and do not darken in the sun. Freckles have normal basal-layer melanocyte numbers but increased melanin. Lentigines have an *increased* number of melanocytes.

Freckles are common, especially in red-haired children. Lentigines may develop in childhood but are more common in a sun-exposed elderly

skin. Freckles require no treatment. Lentigines respond to cryotherapy.

CHLOASMA (MELASMA)

Chloasma is a patterned macular facial pigmentation occurring with pregnancy and in women on oral contraceptives. The pigmentation is symmetrical and often involves the forehead (Fig. 3). Pregnancy stimulates melanocytes generally, and also increases pigmentation of the nipples, lower abdomen and in existing melanocytic naevi. Chloasma improves spontaneously. Sunscreens and camouflage cosmetics can help.

PEUTZ-JEGHERS SYNDROME

Peutz-Jeghers syndrome is a rare autosomal dominant condition. Lentigines around the lips (Fig. 4), buccal mucosa and fingers are associated with small bowel polyps. The polyps may cause intussusception and rarely undergo malignant change.

ADDISON'S DISEASE

Addison's disease is characterized by hypoadrenalism with pituitary overproduction of ACTH. The skin signs are due to excess ACTH, which stimulates melanogenesis. Pigmentation may be generalized or limited to the

Table 3 **Drug-induced pigmentation**

Drug	Effect
Amiodarone	Blue-grey pigmentation of exposed areas
Bleomycin	Diffuse pigmentation, often flexural
Busulphan	Diffuse brown pigment
Chloroquine	Blue-grey pigmentation of face and arms
Chlorpromazine	Slatey-grey pigment in sun-exposed sites
Clofazimine	Red and black pigment
Mepracrine	Yellow (drug deposited)
Minocycline	Blue-black pigment in scars and sun-exposed sites
Psoralens	Topical or systemic photosensitizers (cosmetics)

buccal mucosa (Fig. 5), palmar creases, scars, flexures or areas subjected to friction. Addisonian-like pigmentation is also seen in Cushing's syndrome, hyperthyroidism and acromegaly.

DRUG-INDUCED PIGMENTATION

Drug-induced pigmentation may be due to stimulation of melanogenesis or deposition of the drug in the skin, but often the mechanism is not well understood (Table 3, p. 83).

Table 2 **Causes of hyperpigmentation**

Cause	Example
Drugs	Photosensitizers, psoralens, oestrogens, phenothiazines, minocycline, amiodarone
Endocrine	Addison's disease, chloasma, Cushing's syndrome
Genetic	Racial, freckles, neurofibromatosis, Peutz-Jeghers syndrome
Metabolic	Biliary cirrhosis, haemochromatosis, porphyria
Nutritional	Carotenaemia, malabsorption, malnutrition, pellagra
Post-inflammatory	Eczema, lichen planus, systemic sclerosis, lichen amyloidosis
Other	Acanthosis nigricans, naevi, malignant melanoma, argyria, chronic renal failure

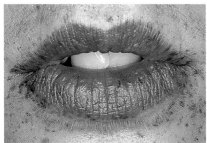
Fig. 4 **The Peutz-Jeghers syndrome showing perioral lentigines.**

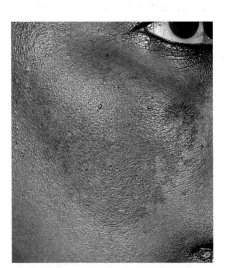
Fig. 3 **Chloasma affecting the cheek and causing a cosmetic disability.**

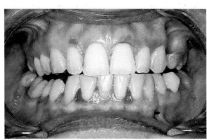
Fig. 5 **Addison's disease, with hyperpigmentation of the gingival and labial mucosa.**

> ### Disorders of pigmentation
>
> - *Vitiligo:* common, autoimmune; well-defined depigmented macules.
> - *Albinism:* rare, autosomal recessive; lack of skin and eye pigment; risk of skin cancer.
> - *Phenylketonuria:* autosomal recessive enzyme defect; fair skin and hair.
> - *Freckles:* brown macules; normal number of melanocytes.
> - *Lentigines:* brown macules; melanocyte numbers increased.
> - *Peutz-Jeghers syndrome:* autosomal dominant disorder of perioral lentigines and intestinal polyps.
> - *Chloasma:* facial pigmentation; related to pregnancy and 'the pill'.
> - *Addison's disease:* ACTH-stimulated melanogenesis of mucosae and flexures.
> - *Drug-induced pigmentation:* due to deposition of pigment or stimulation of melanogenesis.

URTICARIA AND ANGIOEDEMA

Urticaria (hives) is a common eruption characterized by transient, usually pruritic, wheals due to acute dermal oedema from extravascular leakage of plasma. Angioedema signifies a larger area of oedema involving the dermis and subcutis. A classification is shown in Table 1.

AETIOPATHOGENESIS

Urticaria is mediated through immune (allergic) or non-immune mechanisms. Lesions result from the release from mast cells of biologically active substances, particularly histamine, which produce vasodilatation and increased vascular permeability. Several pathways are recognized:

- *IgE-mediated (type I) hypersensitivity* (p. 11) is the best-understood mechanism; antigen cross-links IgE molecules on the surface of the mast cells, resulting in degranulation with release of vasoactive agents.
- *Complement activation* can produce dermal oedema, as in hereditary angioedema or urticaria associated with circulating immune complexes.
- *Direct release of histamine* from mast cells, in a non-immune manner, is caused by some drugs, e.g. opiates and contrast media.
- *Blocking of the prostaglandin pathway* from arachidonic acid, by some drugs such as aspirin and non-steroidal anti-inflammatory agents, promotes urticaria by accumulating vasoactive leukotrienes.
- *A serum histamine-releasing factor* has been suggested in 'chronic' urticaria, although the mechanisms involved in this and in the physical urticarias are poorly understood.

Table 1 **Classification of urticaria and angioedema**

Group	Example
Chronic	Idiopathic
Acute	IgE-mediated, e.g. food allergy, drug reaction
Physical	Dermographism, cholinergic, cold, solar, heat, delayed pressure
Contact	Immune, e.g. animal saliva, or non-immune e.g. nettle sting
Pharmacological	Aspirin, opiates, non-steroidal drugs, food additives
Systemic cause	Systemic LE, lymphoma, thyrotoxicosis, infection, infestation
Inherited	Hereditary angioedema
Other	Urticarial vasculitis, papular (insect bites, p 58), mastocytosis (p. 108), pregnancy (Fig. 5)

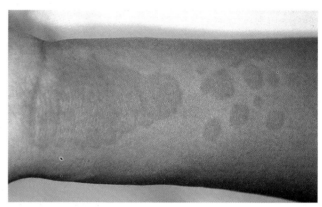

Fig. 1 **Chronic urticaria.** Typical wheals are seen on the forearm.

PATHOLOGY

The dermis is oedematous with dilatation of vessels and mast cell degranulation. Vessel damage and a lymphocytic infiltrate may be seen with urticarial vasculitis.

CLINICAL PRESENTATION

Three-quarters of cases of urticaria fall into the 'chronic idiopathic' or acute categories. Another 20% are due to dermographism, cholinergic urticaria or physical factors. Other causes are rare.

Chronic idiopathic urticaria

Itchy pink wheals appear as papules or plaques anywhere on the skin surface (Fig. 1). Typically they last for less than 24 hours and disappear without a trace. Wheals may be round, annular or polycyclic, and vary in diameter from a few mm to several cm. Their number ranges from a few to many appearing each day, depending on the severity of the condition. Angioedema, usually with swelling of the tongue or lips, may occur (Fig. 2). Pharmacological agents often act as provoking factors, but normally no underlying cause is found. The condition resolves spontaneously within a few months in most cases, although a minority are troubled for years.

Acute urticaria

The sudden onset of urticaria or angioedema may be due to an IgE-mediated type I reaction. The patient often can identify the offending allergen. Commonly it is a food (e.g. egg, fish or peanuts) or a drug (e.g. an antibiotic). Sometimes no cause is found.

Physical urticarias

Cold, heat, sun exposure, pressure and even water can all induce urticaria at the stimulated site. Dermographism, found in 5% of normal people, describes whealing induced by firm stroking of the skin (Fig. 3). In a few individuals it is exaggerated and symptomatic. The wheals in choliner-

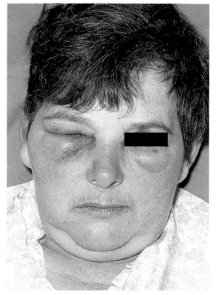

Fig. 2 **Angioedema involving the face.**

gic urticaria are small intensely itchy papules that appear in response to sweating, as induced by exercise, heat, emotion or spicy food. The eruption lasts for a few minutes to an hour.

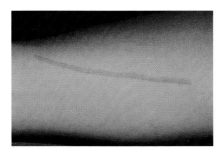

Fig. 3 **Dermographism.** This was caused by stroking the forearm.

Hereditary angioedema

Hereditary angioedema is a rare and potentially fatal autosomal dominant condition. It usually presents in childhood, with episodes of angioedema sometimes involving the larynx (producing respiratory obstruction) and the gastrointestinal tract (causing vomiting and abdominal pain). A deficiency of C_1 esterase inhibitor allows complement activation (e.g. caused by trauma) to go unchecked, with an accumulation of vasoactive mediators. Acute attacks are treated with intravenous infusion of fresh frozen plasma. In the long term, anabolic steroids such as danazol (Danol) are used to promote hepatic synthesis of C_1 esterase inhibitor.

Urticarial vasculitis

Urticarial vasculitis often has an acute onset with widespread urticarial lesions that are unusual as they persist for more than 24 hours and fade leaving purpura (Fig. 4). Systemic abnormalities and low complement levels may be found.

DIFFERENTIAL DIAGNOSIS

Urticaria is usually differentiated from other dermatoses, although pemphigoid (p. 74) or dermatitis herpetiformis (p. 75) occasionally present with an urticarial eruption. Toxic erythema and erythema multiforme (p. 78) may be urticated at first, but when the lesions persist for over 48 hours, urticaria can be excluded. Facial erysipelas sometimes resembles angioedema but has a sharper margin and the patient is unwell with a fever.

INVESTIGATION

Underlying causes or provoking factors are better revealed by a careful history and examination, than by laboratory tests. However, a full blood count, liver function tests, antinuclear factor and urinalysis are often done to exclude systemic conditions (Table 1). Dermographism is demonstrated by firmly stroking the skin, and cold urticaria induced by holding an ice cube on the arm for 1 minute. If congenital angioedema is suspected, the serum C_1 esterase inhibitor level is assayed.

MANAGEMENT

Any underlying cause should be eliminated. Provoking factors, e.g. aspirin ingestion, or swimming (for those with cold urticaria), are to be avoided. Desensitization may be possible for some physical urticarias; for example, individuals with cold urticaria can build up tolerance by gradual immersion of progressively more of the body in cold water. However, the mainstay of treatment is with antihistamines.

Antihistamines

Histamine type 1 receptor blockers (H_1 blockers) reduce the wheal size and the severity of the itch and, given regularly, provide relief. The newer, non-sedative antihistamines, such as terfenadine (Triludan) 60 mg twice daily, astemizole (Hismanal) 10 mg once daily, cetirizine (Zirtek) 10 mg daily or acrivastine (Semprex) 8 mg three times daily, are now preferred unless the sedative qualities of the older preparations are desired. The addition of an H_2 blocker has only a small summative effect if any.

Corticosteroids

Systemic steroids are very occasionally used to control severe acute urticaria or angioedema, and urticarial vasculitis, but are not indicated for chronic urticaria.

Adrenaline

Acute airways obstruction or anaphylactic shock are treated with adrenaline as an intramuscular injection (0.5–1.0 mg: 0.5–1.0 ml of 1/1000), repeated 10 minutes later if necessary. An antihistamine such as chlorpheniramine (Piriton), given by slow intravenous injection, is a useful adjunct. Intravenous steroids are often given, although their onset of action is delayed several hours.

Diet

Salicylates in food aggravate chronic urticaria in up to a third of cases, and dietary azo dyes and benzoic acid preservatives produce an exacerbation in 10%. Diets low in these compounds are tried if routine measures are ineffective.

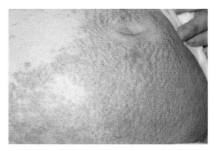

Fig. 5 **An urticated pregnancy-associated eruption.** Often starts in abdominal striae.

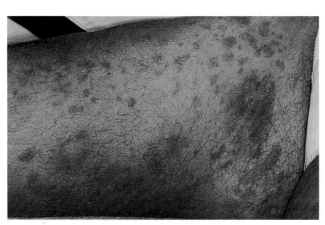

Fig. 4 **Urticarial vasculitis.** Resolving areas have left bruising.

Urticaria

- Urticaria is a common eruption of transient pruritic wheals.
- Associated dermal oedema is usually the result of mast cell degranulation and the release of vasoactive amines.
- No cause is usually found, but urticaria may result from IgE-mediated allergy, physical stimuli, the pharmacological effect of drugs or food additives, or complement deficiencies.
- Causative or provoking factors should be eliminated, and non-sedating antihistamines prescribed.
- Systemic steroids are rarely used in treatment. Aspirin is avoided. Adrenaline is given for anaphylaxis.

BLISTERING DISORDERS

Blistering is often seen with skin disease. It is found with common dermatoses such as acute contact dermatitis, pompholyx, herpes simplex, herpes zoster and bullous impetigo, and it also occurs after insect bites, burns and friction or cold injury. The type of blister depends on the level of cleavage: subcorneal or intraepidermal blisters rupture easily, but subepidermal ones are not so fragile (Fig. 1). The primary bullous disorders, dealt with here, are rare but important.

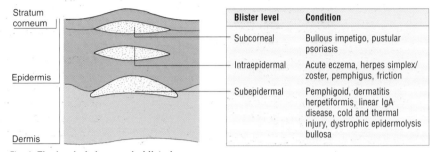

Blister level	Condition
Subcorneal	Bullous impetigo, pustular psoriasis
Intraepidermal	Acute eczema, herpes simplex/zoster, pemphigus, friction
Subepidermal	Pemphigoid, dermatitis herpetiformis, linear IgA disease, cold and thermal injury, dystrophic epidermolysis bullosa

Fig. 1 **The level of cleavage in blistering disorders.**

PEMPHIGUS

Pemphigus is an uncommon, severe and potentially fatal autoimmune blistering disorder affecting the skin and mucous membranes.

Aetiopathogenesis

Ninety per cent of patients have circulating IgG autoantibodies, detectable in the serum by indirect immunofluorescence (p. 119), which bind with an epidermal intercellular cement substance. Adjacent keratinocytes are induced to release proteolytic enzymes which result in loss of adhesion and an intraepidermal split. Direct immunofluorescence (p. 119) shows the inter-cellular deposition of IgG in the suprabasal epidermis. Pemphigus is associated with other organ-specific autoimmune disorders such as myasthenia gravis.

Clinical presentation

In the UK, pemphigus is much less common than pemphigoid and tends to affect middle-aged or young adults. Oral erosions signal the onset of *pemphigus vulgaris* in 50% of patients and often precede cutaneous blistering by months. Flaccid superficial blisters develop over the scalp, face, back, chest and flexures (Fig. 2). The blistering is not always obvious, and lesions may consist of crusted erosions. Untreated, the blistering is progressive and, prior to the introduction of steroids, three out of four patients died within 4 years, usually from uncontrolled fluid and protein loss or secondary infection.

Uncommon variants include *pemphigus foliaceus*, in which shallow erosions appear on the scalp, face and chest, and *pemphigus vegetans*, in which pustular and vegetating lesions

affect the axillae and groins. In Brazil, an endemic form of pemphigus foliaceus, *fogo salvagem*, seems to be due to an infective agent.

Differential diagnosis

Aphthous ulcers or Behçet's disease can simulate the oral erosions of pemphigus. Widespread skin erosions may suggest epidermolysis bullosa or pemphigoid. The diagnosis relies on the histological examination of a bulla, and direct immunofluorescence.

Management

Systemic steroids and other immunosuppressive agents are required. Prednisolone is given initially in a high dose (100–300 mg daily), often with azathioprine or cyclophosphamide. Once blistering is controlled, the steroid dosage can be lowered. Treatment usually needs to be continued

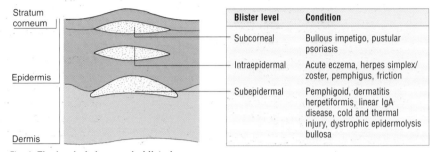

Fig. 2 **Pemphigus vulgaris.** Extensive erosions and flaccid blisters on the trunk.

for years, although remission occasionally occurs. Mortality and morbidity are now more likely to be due to side-effects of the steroid and immunosuppressive therapy than to the disease itself.

PEMPHIGOID

Pemphigoid is a chronic and not uncommon blistering eruption of the elderly.

Aetiopathogenesis

The subepidermal bulla results from the action of enzymes released by inflammatory cells attracted by complement activation, which follows the deposition of IgG antibodies at the basement membrane. The IgG and C_3 are detected by direct immunofluorescence (p. 119). Indirect methods demonstrate circulating autoantibodies in 70% of cases.

Clinical presentation

Bullous pemphigoid usually affects the elderly. Tense large blisters arise on red or normal-looking skin, often of the limbs, trunk and flexures (Fig. 3). Oral lesions occur in only 10% of cases. An urticarial eruption may precede the onset of blistering. Pemphigoid is sometimes localized to one site, often the lower leg. The differential diagnosis of pemphigoid may include dermatitis herpetiformis, linear IgA disease or pemphigus. Immunofluorescence and histology reveal the diagnosis.

Cicatricial pemphigoid mainly affects the ocular and oral mucous membranes. Scarring results and this can cause serious eye problems. *Pemphigoid (herpes) gestationis* is a rare but characteristic bullous eruption associated with pregnancy, which

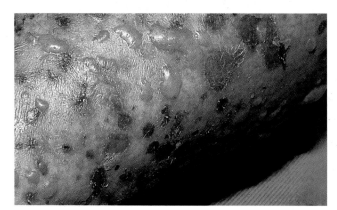

Fig. 3 **Bullous pemphigoid.** Tense blisters on an arm.

remits after the delivery but can recur during subsequent pregnancies.

Management

Pemphigoid responds to a lower dose of steroids than pemphigus: 30–60 mg daily of oral prednisolone are usually sufficient and this can normally be reduced to below 10 mg within weeks. Azathioprine is sometimes also prescribed. The disease is self-limiting in about 50% of cases, and steroids can often be stopped after 2 years. Cicatricial pemphigoid does not respond so well, but pemphigoid gestationis is controlled by standard doses. Steroid-induced side-effects may be a problem, especially in the elderly.

DERMATITIS HERPETIFORMIS

Dermatitis herpetiformis (DH) is an uncommon eruption of symmetrical itchy blisters on the extensor surfaces. Jejunal villus atrophy is an associated finding in most cases.

Aetiopathogenesis

DH is characterized by the finding of granular IgA at the dermal papillae on immunofluorescence, and by the response of the skin lesions (and the villus atrophy seen in over 75% of patients) to a gluten-free diet. Despite this, the cause of the eruption — and its relationship to the undoubted gluten sensitivity of both the gut and the skin — remains unclear. It is doubtful whether the IgA induces the itch, as it is present in asymptomatic patients.

Clinical presentation

DH usually presents in the third or fourth decade and is twice as common in males as in females. The classical onset is with groups of small intensely itchy vesicles on the elbows, knees, buttocks and scalp (Fig. 4). The blisters are often broken by scratching to leave excoriations. Although most patients have small bowel villus atrophy, symptoms of gastrointestinal disturbance and malabsorption are uncommon.

Differential diagnosis

Distinction from scabies, eczema and linear IgA disease is important. Biopsy shows a subepidermal bulla, and direct immunofluorescence of normal-looking skin demonstrates granular IgA at the dermal papilla (p. 119). The small bowel can be investigated by jejunal biopsy. Serum folate, vitamin B_{12} and ferritin estimates detect any biochemical malabsorption. Antiendomysial antibodies are present.

Management

A gluten-free diet is the treatment of choice, as this corrects both the bowel and the skin lesions. Dapsone (50–200 mg daily) will control the eruption and is often given until the gluten-free diet has its beneficial effect. A haemolytic anaemia may occur with dapsone. Regular blood counts are necessary.

LINEAR IgA DISEASE

Linear IgA disease is a rare heterogeneous condition of blisters and urticarial lesions on the back or extensor surfaces (Fig. 5). The disorder responds to dapsone and may resemble DH or pemphigoid. Direct immunofluorescence reveals linear IgA at the basement membrane. The childhood variant shows blistering around the genitalia.

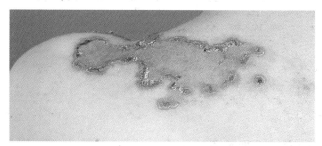

Fig. 5 **Linear IgA disease.** A figurate lesion with peripheral blisters.

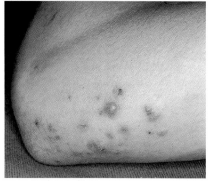

Fig. 4 **Dermatitis herpetiformis.** Itchy blisters on an elbow.

Blistering disorders

Disorder	Clinical details	Direct (and indirect) immunofluorescence	Treatment
Bullous pemphigoid	Not uncommon, seen in elderly, limbs > trunk, oral lesions rare, tense blisters often seen	Linear IgG at basement membrane (indirect: 70% are positive)	Modest dose of oral prednisolone with or without azathioprine
Pemphigus vulgaris	Rare, middle-aged affected, trunk > limbs, often starts with oral lesions, flaccid blisters may be seen	Intercellular epidermal IgG (indirect: 90% are positive)	High dose of oral prednisolone and azathioprine or other immunosuppressive
Dermatitis herpetiformis	Young adults (M > F), extensor surfaces show itchy blisters, villus atrophy is usual	Granular IgA at dermal papilla (indirect: all are negative)	Gluten-free diet with or without dapsone

CONNECTIVE TISSUE DISEASES

The inflammatory disorders of connective tissue often affect several organs, as in systemic lupus erythematosus (LE), but they may also involve the skin alone (e.g. discoid LE). Autoantibodies and cell-mediated immunity against normal cellular components (e.g. nuclei) are a feature of these diseases, which can thus be regarded as 'autoimmune'.

LUPUS ERYTHEMATOSUS

Systemic LE is a serious multisystem disease that involves vascular and connective tissues. *Discoid LE* is a chronic indolent cutaneous disorder of scaly atrophic plaques in sun-exposed sites.

Aetiopathogenesis

Autoantibodies to nuclear, nucleolar and cytoplasmic antigens are found in LE. Over 90% of systemic LE patients have circulating antinuclear antibodies as compared to less than 25% of those with discoid LE. Subjects with systemic LE may also have T suppressor cell dysfunction. UV radiation often brings out the eruption, perhaps by generating nuclear products in the skin. Systemic LE is associated with HLA phenotypes B8 and DR3, and it may be triggered by certain drugs.

Pathology

Discoid lesions show epidermal atrophy, hyperkeratosis and basal

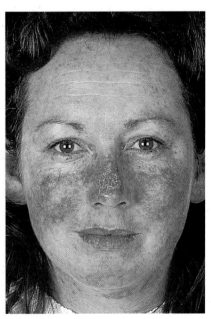

Fig. 1 **Systemic LE.** The typical butterfly eruption is present on the face.

layer degeneration. Systemic lesions have similar changes with dermal oedema, inflammatory infiltrate and sometimes vasculitis. Direct immunofluorescence shows a 'lupus band' of immunoglobulins and complement at the dermo-epidermal junction of the lesional and normal sun-exposed skin in systemic LE, and of lesional skin in discoid LE.

Clinical presentation

Systemic LE

Skin signs are found in 75%. The facial butterfly eruption (Fig. 1) is well known, but photosensitivity, discoid lesions, diffuse alopecia and vasculitis also occur. Multisystem involvement with serological or haematological abnormalities must be demonstrated to diagnose systemic LE (Table 1). The female: male ratio is 8:1.

Table 1 **Organ involvement in systemic LE**

Organ	Involvement
Skin	Photosensitivity, facial rash, vasculitis, hair loss
Blood	Anaemia, thrombocytopenia
Joints	Arthritis, tenosynovitis
Kidney	Glomerulonephritis
Heart	Pericarditis, endocarditis
CNS	Psychosis, infarction
Lungs	Pneumonitis, effusion

Discoid LE

One or more round or oval plaques appear on the face, scalp or hands (Fig. 2). The lesions are well-demarcated, red, atrophic, scaly and show keratin plugs in dilated follicles. Scarring leaves alopecia on the scalp and hypopigmentation in those with a pigmented skin. Remission occurs in 40%. Internal involvement is not a feature, and only 5% develop systemic LE. Women outnumber men by 2:1.

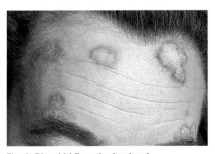

Fig. 2 **Discoid LE on the forehead.**

Other forms

Subacute cutaneous LE is characterized by widespread symmetrical scaly plaques on sun-exposed sites of the face and forearms. Internal disease may occur, and anti-Ro antibodies are found. *Neonatal LE* is due to the placental transfer of anti-Ro antibodies from affected mothers to their neonates, who develop an annular atrophic eruption, sometimes with heart block.

Differential diagnosis

Discoid LE can usually be differentiated from other facial rashes such as rosacea, seborrhoeic dermatitis, lupus vulgaris or psoriasis. A biopsy should be performed. The photosensitive eruption of systemic LE may resemble polymorphic light eruption, dermatomyositis or drug reaction. Skin biopsy, with immunofluorescence, is helpful.

Management

Discoid LE usually responds to potent or very potent topical steroids which, in this instance, can be applied to the face. Sunblock creams are helpful. Widespread disease may need systemic therapy with chloroquine: the risk of retinopathy demands regular ophthalmological checks. The treatment of systemic LE depends on the type of involvement. Sunscreens reduce photosensitivity, but if there is internal disease, systemic steroids are required, often with immunosuppressive agents.

SYSTEMIC SCLEROSIS

Systemic sclerosis is an uncommon, progressive multisystem disease in which collagen deposition and fibrosis occur in several organs.

Aetiopathogenesis

Most patients have circulating antibodies to nuclear, nucleolar or cytoplasmic antigens, but their importance is unclear. Endothelial cell damage is central and leads to inflammation and fibrosis. T cell factors may be involved. Immunofluorescence shows immunoglobulin and complement at the dermo-epidermal junction.

Clinical presentation

Raynaud's phenomenon (p. 66) is frequently the presenting sign. The skin

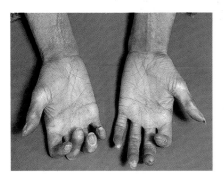

Fig. 3 **Systemic sclerosis.** Note the tightly bound waxy skin on the fingers (sclerodactyly) and resorption of the finger pulps.

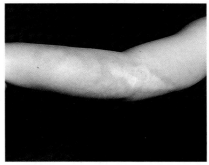

Fig. 4 **Morphoea.** Seen here on the arm of a child. The white indurated plaque has an erythematous edge.

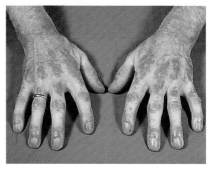

Fig. 5 **Dermatomyositis.** A streaky eruption is seen on the dorsal aspects of the hands.

of the fingers, forearms, and lower legs becomes tight, waxy and stiff, and the finger pulps are resorbed (Fig. 3). Facial signs include perioral furrowing, telangiectasia (p. 107) and restricted mouth opening. Internal organ involvement, e.g. renal failure, may prove fatal (Table 2). Women are affected more than men (F:M 4:1). The diagnosis is rarely in doubt, although chronic graft-versus-host disease shows similar changes. In the CREST syndrome, a variant with a better prognosis, involvement is confined to *C*alcinosis, *R*aynaud's phenomenon, o*E*sophageal dysmotility, *S*clerodactyly and *T*elangiectasia.

Table 2 **Organ involvement in systemic sclerosis**

Organ	Involvement
Skin	Raynaud's phenomenon, calcinosis, sclerodactyly, telangiectasia
Gut	Oesophageal dysmotility, malabsorption
Lung	Fibrosis, cyst formation
Heart	Pericarditis, myocardial fibrosis
Kidney	Renal failure, hypertension
Muscle	Myositis

Management

Treatment is mainly supportive. Nifedipine can help Raynaud's phenomenon. Systemic steroids, penicillamine and immunosuppressives have been used with little benefit. Photophoresis may be tried (p. 107).

MORPHOEA (LOCALIZED SCLERODERMA)

Morphoea consists of localized indurated plaques or bands of sclerosis on the skin. Internal disease is not found. The cause is unknown, although it may follow trauma. Histology shows bands of collagen with loss of appendages.

Morphoea presents with round or oval plaques of induration and erythema, often with a purplish edge (Fig. 4). These become shiny and white, eventually leaving atrophic hairless pigmented patches. The trunk or proximal limbs are affected. Morphoea is more common in women (F:M 3:1). *Linear morphoea* may involve the face or a limb and, when seen in a child, can retard growth of the underlying tissues, including bone. A rare, *generalized form* may encase the trunk but avoids the hands and feet.

There is no established treatment, although topical steroids are often given. The disease usually resolves spontaneously within a few months.

DERMATOMYOSITIS

Dermatomyositis is an uncommon disorder in which inflammation of skin and muscle gives a distinctive eruption, with muscle weakness of varying severity.

Clinical presentation

In dermatomyositis/polymyositis, skin changes or muscle weakness may predominate, and underlying malignancy is found in a subgroup. The cause is unknown, but autoimmune mechanisms are proposed. The typical eruption is a lilac-blue discoloration around the eyelids, cheeks and forehead, often with oedema. Bluish-red papules or streaks on the dorsal aspects of the hands (Fig. 5), elbows and knees are seen, sometimes with pigmentation and nail fold telangiectasia. Photosensitivity is common. An association with malignancy exists in patients over 40 years, 40% of whom have an underlying tumour, usually of the lung, breast or stomach. A childhood variant mainly affects the muscles and causes calcinosis and contractures.

Management

Investigations must define the degree of myositis and, in the middle-aged or elderly, exclude the possibility of underlying neoplasia. Treatment is with systemic steroids in moderate doses, often with an immunosuppressive such as azathioprine. Immunoglobulin infusion is under evaluation (p. 107).

Connective tissue diseases

- *Systemic LE* is an autoimmune, multisystem disease in which a butterfly rash, photosensitivity, vasculitis and alopecia may be seen.
- *Discoid LE* is confined to the skin. Scaly atrophic plaques and scarring alopecia are found. Topical steroids and sunscreens are helpful.
- *Systemic sclerosis* is a serious multisystem disorder. Sclerodactyly, Raynaud's phenomenon, telangiectasia and calcinosis are seen.
- *Morphoea* is characterized by white indurated plaques, usually on the trunk and proximal limbs. In children it may retard growth of underlying tissues, producing atrophy. In adults the condition is generally self-limiting.
- *Dermatomyositis* is an autoimmune inflammation of skin and muscle. The skin signs are a lilac-blue discoloration around the eyelids and red streaks on the dorsa of the hands. Exclude underlying malignancy in those over 40.

VASCULITIS AND THE REACTIVE ERYTHEMAS

Vasculitis and the reactive erythemas are characterized by inflammation within or around blood vessels. This may result from a type III hypersensitivity response, with circulating immune complexes, but other mechanisms are also possible.

VASCULITIS

Vasculitis is a disease process usually centred on small or medium-sized blood vessels. It is often due to circulating immune complexes (CIC).

Aetiopathogenesis

The CIC, which may be associated with several conditions (Table 1), lodge in the vessel wall where they activate complement, attract polymorphs and damage tissue. Inflammatory cells infiltrate vessels. Endothelial cells may show swelling, fibrinoid change or necrosis.

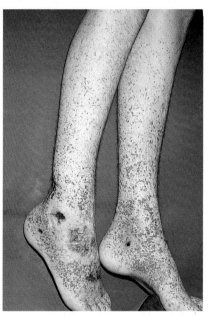

Fig. 1 **Vasculitis with purpura and impending skin necrosis.**

Table 1 **Causes of vasculitis**

Group	Example
Idiopathic	50% of cases
Blood disease	Cryoglobulinaemia
Connective tissue disease	Systemic LE, rheumatoid arthritis
Drugs	Sulphonamides, penicillin, serum sickness
Infections	Hepatitis B, streptococci, M. leprae, Rickettsia
Neoplasia	Lymphoma, leukaemia
Other	Wegener's granulomatosis, giant cell arteritis, polyarteritis nodosa

Clinical presentation

This depends on the size and site of vessels involved. Vasculitis may be confined to the skin, or may be systemic and involve the joints, kidneys, lungs, gut and nervous system. The skin signs are of palpable purpura, often painful and usually on the lower legs or buttocks (Fig. 1).

- *Henoch-Schönlein purpura* describes these signs, with arthritis, abdominal pain and haematuria. It is a small vessel vasculitis which mainly affects children and often follows a streptococcal infection.
- *Nodular vasculitis*, characterized by tender subcutaneous nodules on the lower legs, results when deeper dermal vessels are involved.

- *Polyarteritis nodosa* is characterized by a necrotizing vasculitis in medium-sized arteries. It is uncommon and afflicts middle-aged men who, in addition to tender subcutaneous nodules along the line of arteries, may develop hypertension, renal failure and neuropathy.
- *Wegener's granulomatosis* is a rare but potentially fatal granulomatous vasculitis of unknown cause. Malaise, upper respiratory tract necrosis, glomerulonephritis, lung involvement and, in 50% of cases, a cutaneous vasculitis are found.
- *Giant cell arteritis* affects medium-sized arteries in the elderly. Visual loss may result if prednisolone is withheld. Patients present with scalp tenderness due to temporal artery involvement which can progress to scalp necrosis.

In vasculitis, a skin biopsy is helpful along with tests to look for internal organ involvement. Other causes of purpura need exclusion.

Management

The cause is identified and remedied if possible. Many idiopathic cases settle with bed rest but, if lesions continue to develop and if internal organs are involved, treatment is indicated. Dapsone, 100 mg daily, is often effec-

tive for cutaneous vasculitis. Otherwise, prednisolone (sometimes with an immunosuppressive) is prescribed. Giant cell arteritis, polyarteritis nodosa and Wegener's granulomatosis nearly always require oral steroids and immunosuppression.

ERYTHEMA MULTIFORME

Erythema multiforme is an immune-mediated disease, characterized by target lesions on the hands and feet. It has a variety of causes.

Aetiopathogenesis

CIC, which result from a number of causes (Table 2), are deposited in blood vessels. Cell-mediated immunity may be involved. No provoking factor is found in 50% of cases. On histology, the epidermis is necrotic and the dermis shows oedema, an inflammatory infiltrate and vasodilatation.

Table 2 **Causes of erythema multiforme**

Group	Cause
Idiopathic	50% of cases
Viral	Herpes simplex, hepatitis B, orf, Mycoplasma
Bacterial	Streptococci
Fungal	Coccidioidomycosis
Drugs	Penicillin, barbiturate, sulphonamide
Other	LE, pregnancy, malignancy

Clinical presentation

Typical target lesions, seen on the hands and feet, consist of red rings with central pale or purple areas which may blister (Fig. 2). Involvement of the oral, conjunctival and genital mucosae is not uncommon and, if extreme, is known as the *Stevens-Johnson syndrome*. Crops of new lesions appear for 2–3 weeks. The

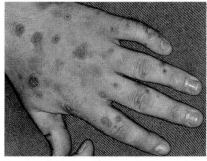

Fig. 2 **Erythema multiforme.** Target lesions are seen here on the dorsal aspect of the hand.

differential diagnosis includes toxic erythema (p. 82), toxic epidermal necrolysis, Sweet's disease, urticaria or pemphigoid. A biopsy is often helpful. *Toxic epidermal necrolysis* (p. 83) may sometimes represent erythema multiforme in a severe form.

Management
Identification and treatment of the underlying cause is the ideal. Mild cases resolve spontaneously and require symptomatic measures only. Extensive involvement necessitates hospital admission for supportive therapy. Systemic steroids are often prescribed to moderate the acute symptoms, although it is debatable whether they affect the outcome.

ERYTHEMA NODOSUM
Erythema nodosum is a panniculitis (i.e. an inflammation of the subcutaneous fat) that usually presents as painful red nodules on the lower legs. It is believed to result from CIC deposition in vessels of the subcutis. Infection, drugs and some systemic diseases are underlying causes (Table 3).

Table 3 **Causes of erythema nodosum**

Group	Cause
Idiopathic	About 20% of cases
Bacterial	Streptococci, TB, leprosy, *Yersinia*, *Mycoplasma*, *Rickettsia*
Fungal	Coccidioidomycosis
Viral	Cat-scratch fever
Drugs	Sulphonamides, oral contraceptives
Systemic diseases	Inflammatory bowel disease, sarcoidosis, Behçet's disease, malignancy (rare)

Clinical presentation
Deep, firm and tender reddish-blue nodules, 1–5 cm in diameter, develop on the calves (Fig. 3), shins and occasionally on the forearms. Joint pains and fever are common. Spontaneous resolution usually occurs within 8 weeks. Women are affected more than men (F:M 3:1). Other causes of panniculitis (e.g. pancreatic disease, cold, trauma and LE), cellulitis and phlebitis need to be excluded. If TB or sarcoidosis are suspected, a chest radiograph, Mantoux test or Kviem test are indicated.

Management
As spontaneous remission is usual, active therapy is rarely needed, although a non-steroidal anti-

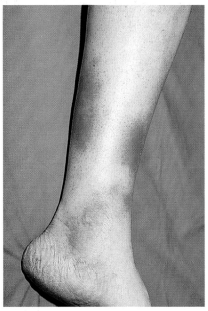
Fig. 3 **Erythema nodosum of the lower leg.**

inflammatory such as ibuprofen or indomethacin may help.

SWEET'S DISEASE
Sweet's disease (*acute febrile neutrophilic dermatosis*) occurs as raised plum-coloured plaques on the face or limbs (Fig. 4) with, typically, fever and a raised neutrophil count. It is not

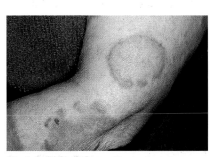
Fig. 4 **Sweet's disease.** Shown here is a variant associated with rheumatoid arthritis. Infiltrated annular plaques are seen on the arm.

a true vasculitis but results from polymorph infiltration of the dermis. Leukaemia, ulcerative colitis and other disorders may be associated and must be excluded. Treatment with prednisolone is usually needed.

GRAFT-VERSUS-HOST (GVH) DISEASE
GVH disease occurs when immunologically competent donor lymphocytes react against host tissues, principally the skin and gut. It is mostly found with bone marrow transplant, e.g. given for leukaemia or aplastic anaemia. Fever, malaise and a morbilliform eruption (Fig. 5) which may progress to toxic epidermal necrolysis, typify the acute GVH reaction. Chronic GVH disease may resemble lichen planus or systemic sclerosis. A skin biopsy often helps and treatment with systemic steroids is usually needed.

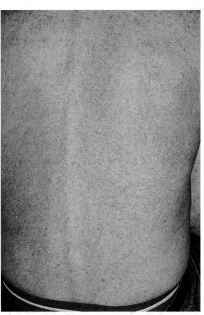
Fig. 5 **Graft-versus-host disease.** An acute eruption is shown in a patient following bone-marrow transplant.

Vasculitis and the reactive erythemas
- *Vasculitis* is a CIC disorder showing palpable purpura, sometimes with internal organ involvement. Investigations may reveal the underlying cause.
- *Erythema multiforme* is an immune-mediated reaction with target and mucosal lesions, often due to infection or drugs.
- *Erythema nodosum* presents as painful deep nodules on the lower legs and is regarded as a CIC response to infection, drugs or internal disease.
- *Sweet's disease* is characterized by plum-coloured plaques on the face and limbs. Leukaemia or a systemic disorder may be associated.

SKIN CHANGES IN INTERNAL CONDITIONS

Skin signs are seen with many internal disorders and are not uncommonly their presenting feature. The astute dermatologist can therefore recognize hitherto undiagnosed systemic disease.

SKIN SIGNS OF ENDOCRINE AND METABOLIC DISEASE

Almost all endocrine diseases (and several metabolic defects) have cutaneous signs which depend on the over- or under-production of a hormone or metabolite (Table 1).

DIABETES MELLITUS

C. albicans or bacterial infection is more common with untreated or poorly controlled diabetes. The neuropathy or arteriopathy of diabetes may result in *ulcers* on the feet (p. 69), and an associated secondary hyperlipidaemia can produce *eruptive xanthomas* (Fig. 4). *Diabetic dermopathy* describes depressed pigmented scars on the shins, associated with diabetic microangiopathy. *Necrobiosis lipoidica* (Fig. 1), characterized by shiny atrophic yellowish-red plaques on the shins, is in 70% of cases found in diabetics or in those who later develop the disease, although it affects less than 1% of all diabetics. Histologically, degenerate dermal collagen is seen with epithelioid cells and giant cells. The condition is chronic, and may ulcerate. It is unresponsive to treatment. In contrast, *granuloma annu-*

Table 1 **Skin signs of endocrine and metabolic disorders**

Disorders	Skin signs
Diabetes mellitus	Necrobiosis lipoidica, granuloma annulare, xanthomas, *C. albicans* infection, 'dermopathy', neuropathic ulcers
Thyrotoxicosis	Pink soft skin, hyperhidrosis, alopecia, pigmentation, onycholysis, clubbing, pretibial myxoedema, palmar erythema
Myxoedema	Alopecia (including eyebrows), coarse hair, dry puffy yellowish skin (e.g. hands, face), asteatotic eczema, xanthomas
Addison's disease	Pigmentation (p. 71), vitiligo, axillary and pubic hair loss
Cushing's disease	Pigmentation, hirsutism, striae, acne, obesity, buffalo 'hump'
Acromegaly	Thickened moist greasy skin, pigmentation, skin tags
Phenylketonuria	Fair hair and skin, atopic eczema (p. 70)
Hyperlipidaemia	Xanthomas, xanthelasma
Cutaneous porphyrias	Photosensitivity, blistering, skin fragility, atrophic scarring, hypertrichosis, pigmentation (p. 42)

lare — recognized as palpable annular lesions on the hands, feet or face (Fig. 2) — is only rarely associated with diabetes and usually fades in 12 months. It must be differentiated from tinea corporis.

THYROID DISEASE

Both over- and under-production of thyroxine result in skin and hair changes (Table 1). *Pretibial myxoedema* (Fig. 3), seen in patients with hyperthyroidism, presents on the shins as raised erythematous plaques due to the deposition of mucin in the dermis. Topical steroids may be of benefit.

HYPERLIPIDAEMIA

Both primary (genetic metabolic defects) and secondary (associated with diabetes, hypothyroidism or the nephrotic syndrome) lipid abnormalities may produce a variety of xanthomatous deposits. These may be:

- *eruptive* — red-yellow papules; shoulders, buttocks (Fig. 4)
- *tendinous* — subcutaneous nodules; hand, foot, or Achilles tendons
- *plane* — yellow-orange macules in palmar creases
- *tuberous* — yellow-orange nodules on knees and elbows.

Xanthelasma, seen as yellowish plaques on the eyelids, are not always due to a lipid abnormality. Treatment of xanthomas is usually aimed at the underlying hyperlipidaemia.

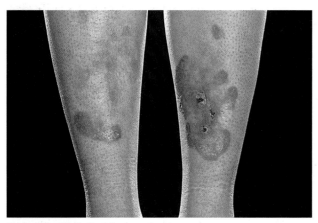

Fig. 1 **Necrobiosis lipoidica.** Yellowish-red atrophic areas are seen on the shins of a diabetic.

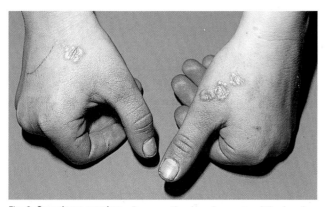

Fig. 2 **Granuloma annulare.** Seen on the dorsal aspects of the hands.

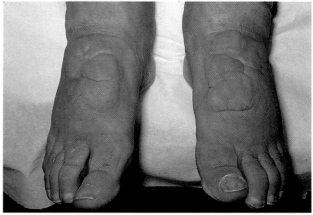

Fig. 3 **Pretibial myxoedema.** The patient had been thyrotoxic.

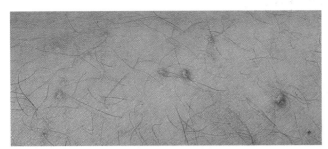

Fig. 4 **Eruptive xanthomas.** The patient had recently presented with diabetes mellitus.

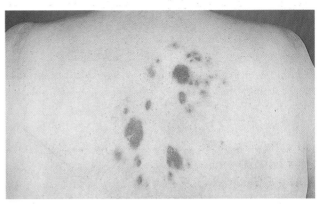

Fig. 5 **Sarcoidosis.** Plum-coloured plaques are seen here on the upper back.

SKIN SIGNS OF NUTRITIONAL AND OTHER INTERNAL DISORDERS

Skin changes are common with nutritional deficiency and are not infrequent with gastrointestinal, hepatic and renal disease.

NUTRITIONAL DEFICIENCY

Protein malnutrition results in retarded growth, wasted muscles, oedema and skin changes of altered pigmentation, desquamation, ulcers with (in Black Africans) dry and pale-brown/red hair. *Vitamin C deficiency* (scurvy) and *niacin deficiency* (pellagra) produce distinct lesions. In the UK, scurvy is mainly seen in elderly men who do not eat fresh fruit or vegetables. Deficiencies of other B vitamins and of iron also produce cutaneous changes (Table 2). *Acrodermatitis enteropathica* is a rare inherited defect of zinc absorption seen in weaned infants and cured by zinc supplements.

GASTROINTESTINAL DISEASE

Malabsorption and its deficiency states have accompanying skin problems that include dryness, eczema, ichthyosis, pigmentation and defects of the hair and nails. Some gut disorders show specific skin changes (Table 2). *Coeliac disease* is associated with an eczema (in addition to the link of dermatitis herpetiformis with gluten enteropathy, p. 75). and both *Crohn's disease* and *ulcerative colitis* induce various eruptions. *Peutz-Jeghers syndrome* (p. 71) and *pseudoxan-*

thoma elasticum (p. 89) affect both the skin and the gut. *Bowel by-pass surgery* induces a vesiculopustular eruption.

OTHER INTERNAL DISORDERS

Hepatic and *renal disease* often produce troublesome itching and pigmentation. Lesions may also be related to the underlying disease process, e.g. primary biliary cirrhosis (associated with systemic sclerosis) or vasculitis.

Sarcoidosis, a disorder of unknown aetiology in which granulomas develop commonly in the lungs, lymph nodes, bone and nervous tissue, affects the skin in a third of cases. Cutaneous changes are variable and include brownish-red papules (typically on the face), nodules, plaques (on the limbs and shoulders, Fig. 5) and scar involvement. *Lupus pernio* is a particular pattern of sarcoidosis which appears as dusky-red infiltrated plaques on the nose or, occasionally, the fingers. *Erythema nodosum* may also result. Topical steroids have little effect. Resistant lesions may improve with intralesional steroid injection, but oral prednisolone or methotrexate is sometimes prescribed, particularly when there is progressive internal disease.

SKIN CHANGES IN PREGNANCY

Skin changes are common in pregnancy. Pigmentation generally increases (p. 71), melanocytic naevi become more prominent and spider naevi and abdominal striae develop. Telogen effluvium may occur in the postpartum period (p. 62). Pruritus and an urticated papular eruption (p. 73) are not uncommon, though pemphigoid gestationis (p. 75) is rare. The effect on common dermatoses is variable and unpredictable: psoriasis tends to improve, but eczema may get worse.

Table 2 **Skin signs of nutritional and internal disorders**

Disorder	Skin signs
Protein malnutrition	Pigmentation, dry skin, oedema, pale-brown/orange hair
Iron deficiency	Alopecia, koilonychia, itching, angular cheilitis
Scurvy	Perifollicular purpura, bleeding gums, woody oedema
Pellagra	Light-exposed dermatitis and pigmentation
Acrodermatitis enteropathica	Perianal/perioral red scaly pustular eruption in infants, failure to thrive, diarrhoea, poor wound healing
Malabsorption	Dry itchy skin, ichthyosis, eczema, oedema
Liver disease	Pruritus, spider naevi, palmar erythema, white nails, pigmentation, xanthomas, porphyria cutanea tarda, zinc deficiency
Renal failure	Pruritus, pigmentation, white/red nails, dry skin with fine scaling
Pancreatic disease	Panniculitis, thrombophlebitis, glucagonoma syndrome
Crohn's disease	Perianal abscesses, sinuses, fistulae, erythema nodosum, Sweet's disease, aphthous stomatitis, glossitis
Ulcerative colitis	Pyoderma gangrenosum, erythema nodosum, Sweet's disease
Sarcoidosis	Nodules, plaques, erythema nodosum, dactylitis, lupus pernio, scar granulomas, small papules, nail involvement

Skin changes in internal conditions

- Endocrine and metabolic disorders, nutritional deficiencies and malabsorption are frequently associated with skin changes.
- Liver and kidney failure particularly are complicated by pruritus and pigmentation.
- Inflammatory bowel disease and sarcoidosis have specific skin manifestations, often granulomatous or with cellular infiltration.

DRUG ERUPTIONS

Reactions to drugs are common and often produce an eruption. Almost any drug can result in any reaction, although some patterns are more common with certain drugs. Not all reactions are 'allergic' in nature.

AETIOPATHOGENESIS

Drug-induced skin reactions have several possible mechanisms:

- *excessive therapeutic effect,* e.g. purpura resulting from accidental overdosage with anticoagulants
- *pharmacological side-effects,* e.g. dry lips and nasal mucosa with isotretinoin or bone marrow suppression by cytotoxics
- *modulation of the immune response,* e.g. a type IV skin reaction in leprosy when cell-mediated immunity improves following drug therapy
- *deposition* of the drug (or metabolites) in the skin, e.g. gold
- *idiosyncratic reaction* peculiar to that individual
- *facilitative effect,* e.g. when antibiotics suppress the normal skin flora, or drugs exacerbate psoriasis
- *immune hypersensitivity* in any of the four types (p. 11).

CLINICAL PRESENTATION

Drug eruptions present in many guises and come into the differential diagnosis of several rashes. When suspected, it is vital to obtain a detailed history of all the drugs taken over the preceding 2 or 3 weeks. This must include 'over the counter' preparations (e.g. for headaches or constipation) not normally regarded as 'drugs' by the patient. In subjects taking several preparations, a drug introduced during a two week period before the eruption starts must be viewed as the most likely culprit, although a reaction may occur to a drug taken safely for years. The majority of drug eruptions fit into a defined category (Table 1). The most common and characteristic ones are outlined below. Other patterns, e.g. lichenoid, photosensitive, pigmentation and erythroderma, have been mentioned previously.

Toxic erythema

Toxic erythema, the commonest type of drug eruption may be *morbilliform* (measles-like) or *urticarial,* or may resemble *erythema multiforme.* It usually affects the trunk more than the extremities (Fig. 1), and may be accompanied by fever or followed by

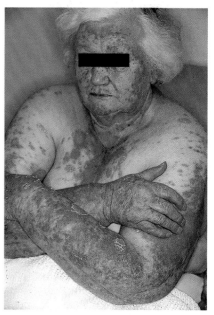

Fig. 1 **Toxic erythema.** This morbilliform variant was due to chlorpropamide.

peeling of the skin. Drugs commonly implicated include ampicillin, sulphonamides and carbamazepine. It is also caused by scarlet fever (group A streptococci) or viral infections. The eruption clears 1-2 weeks after stopping the offending drug.

Table 1 **Patterns of drug eruptions**

Drug eruption	Description	Drugs commonly responsible
Acneiform	Like acne: papulopustules, no comedones	Androgens, bromides, dantrolene, isoniazid, lithium, phenobarbitone, quinidine, steroids
Bullous	Various types; some phototoxic, some 'fixed'	Barbiturates (overdose), frusemide, nalidixic acid (phototoxic), penicillamine (pemphigus-like)
Eczematous	Not common; seen when topical sensitization is followed by systemic treatment	Neomycin, penicillin, sulphonamide, ethylenediamine (cross-reacts with aminophylline), benzocaine (cross reacts with chlorpropamide), parabens, allopurinol
Erythema multiforme	Target lesions (p. 78)	Sulphonamides, phenytoin, penicillins, ACE inhibitors, calcium-channel blockers
Erythroderma	Exfoliative dermatitis'(p. 40)	Allopurinol, captopril, carbamazepine, diltiazem, gold, isoniazid, phenytoin, sulphonamides
Fixed drug eruption	Round red-purple plaques recur at same site	Ibuprofen, phenolphthalein, paracetamol, quinine, sulphonamides, tetracyclines
Hair loss	Telogen effluvium (p. 62) Anagen effluvium (p. 62)	Anticoagulants, bezafibrate, carbimazole, oral contraceptive pill Cytotoxics, acitretin
Hypertrichosis	Excess vellus hair growth (p. 63)	Minoxidil, cyclosporin, phenytoin, corticosteroids, androgens
Lupus erythematosus	LE-like syndrome (p. 76)	Hydralazine, isoniazid, penicillamine, phenytoin, procainamide, beta-blockers
Lichenoid	Like lichen planus (p. 36)	Beta-blockers, captopril, gold, isoniazid, PAS, quinine, penicillamine, thiazides
Photosensitive	Sun-exposed sites, may blister or pigment (p. 83, Fig. 4)	Non-steroidal anti-inflammatories, ACE inhibitors, amiodarone, thiazides, tetracyclines
Pigmentation	Melanin or drug-deposition (p. 83, Fig. 5)	Amiodarone, bleomycin, psoralens, chlorpromazine, minocycline, antimalarials
Psoriasiform	Psoriasis-like appearance (see text)	Beta-blockers, gold, methyl dopa: lithium and antimalarials exacerbate psoriasis
Toxic epidermal necrolysis	Scalded skin appearance (see text)	Allopurinol, barbiturate, phenytoin, non-steroidal anti-inflammatories, penicillins, sulphonamides
Toxic erythema	Commonest pattern (see text)	Antibiotics (notably ampicillin), gold, sulphonamides, thiazides, allopurinol, carbamazepine
Urticaria	Many mechanisms (p. 72)	ACE inhibitors, penicillins, opiates, salicylates, X-ray contrast media, vaccines
Vasculitis	Immune complex reaction	Allopurinol, captopril, penicillins, phenytoin, sulphonamides, thiazides

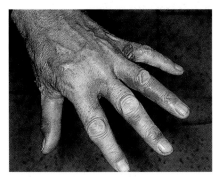

Fig. 2 **Fixed drug eruption.** The typical dusky erythematous lesions, some of which are bullous, followed the ingestion of phenolphthalein in an over-the-counter laxative.

Fixed drug eruption

This specific but uncommon eruption is characterized by round red or purplish plaques (Fig. 2) that recur at the same site each time the causative agent is taken. The lesions may blister and leave pigmentation on clearing. Quinine, phenolphthalein (in laxatives) and sulphonamides are often responsible.

Toxic epidermal necrolysis

Toxic epidermal necrolysis, a serious and life-threatening eruption, is a drug-induced adult disorder similar to *staphylococcal scalded skin syndrome* of childhood (p. 45). The skin is red, swollen and separates as in a scald (Fig. 3). The split is intraepidermal. Mucosal lesions are usual, and the condition may on occasions be a severe form of erythema multiforme. The extensive skin loss results in problems of fluid and electrolyte balance, as seen with extensive burns, and the patient must be managed in an intensive care unit. Drugs which commonly cause this condition

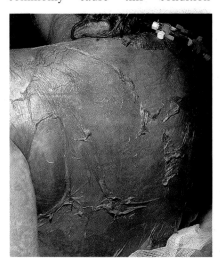

Fig. 3 **Toxic epidermal necrolysis.** The damaged epidermis has sheared off to leave extensive areas of eroded skin.

include non-steroidal anti-inflammatories, allopurinol, sulphonamides and phenytoin.

Psoriasiform and bullous eruptions

Drugs such as lithium or chloroquine can exacerbate existing psoriasis. Other agents, including beta-blockers, gold and methyl dopa, may provoke a psoriasis-like eruption.

Fixed drug eruption, phototoxic reaction, drug-induced pemphigus and barbiturate overdosage (at pressure sites) may all blister (Table 1).

DIFFERENTIAL DIAGNOSIS

The exact differential diagnosis depends on the type of drug eruption. A typical morbilliform rash occurring a few days after antibiotic therapy usually presents no diagnostic difficulties, but could be confused with a toxic erythema associated with the infection for which the antibiotic was prescribed. The situation is more complicated when an eruption occurs in

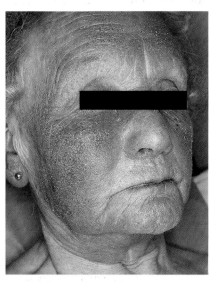

Fig. 4 **Photosensitivity.** This was caused by taking a thiazide diuretic.

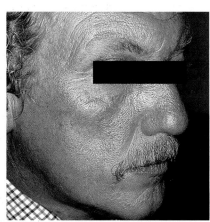

Fig. 5 **Pigmentation.** This was due to treatment with amiodarone.

an ill patient treated with a multiplicity of drugs. The determination of which drug is responsible depends on accurate prescribing records and a knowledge of the potential of each drug for causing a reaction. Table 2 shows the types of eruption seen with some of the more commonly prescribed drugs. Laboratory and skin tests are generally unhelpful in diagnosing a drug eruption.

MANAGEMENT

Withdrawal of the offending drug usually leads to clearance of the eruption within 2 or so weeks. Simple emollients or topical steroids can help to ease the eruption until it resolves. Patients should be given advice about which drugs they must avoid. Provocation tests to confirm that a drug has been culpable are not recommended because of the possibility of inducing a severe reaction.

Table 2 **Eruptions seen with some commonly prescribed drugs**

Drug	Eruption
ACE inhibitors	Pruritus, urticaria, toxic erythema
Antibiotics	Toxic erythema, urticaria, fixed drug eruption, erythema multiforme
Beta-blockers	Psoriasiform, Raynaud's phenomenon, lichenoid eruption
Non-steroidal anti-inflammatories	Toxic erythema, erythroderma, toxic epidermal necrolysis
Oral contraceptive	Chloasma, alopecia, acne, candidiasis
Phenothiazines	Photosensitivity, pigmentation
Thiazides	Toxic erythema, photosensitivity, lichenoid eruption, vasculitis

Drug eruptions

- Drug reactions may be pharmacological or idiosyncratic, as well as immune-mediated.
- Drugs which commonly cause drug eruptions are *ampicillin, ACE inhibitors, sulphonamides, thiazides* and *non-steroidal anti-inflammatories.*
- The commonest pattern is *toxic erythema*, often morbilliform.
- The most severe involvement is *toxic epidermal necrolysis*, which may be fatal.
- A drug eruption typically begins within 3 days of starting a drug (if it has been taken before) and clears about 2 weeks after stopping it.
- Withdrawal of the drug and avoidance of related compounds are necessary.

ASSOCIATIONS WITH MALIGNANCY

Internal malignancy causes a variety of skin changes (Table 1). Apart from direct infiltration, the mechanisms of these effects are poorly understood.

CONDITIONS ASSOCIATED WITH MALIGNANCY

The following rare skin eruptions are characteristic and strongly indicate an underlying malignancy:

- acanthosis nigricans
- erythema gyratum repens
- necrolytic migratory erythema
- Paget's disease
- extra-mammary Paget's disease
- skin secondaries.

ACANTHOSIS NIGRICANS

Acanthosis nigricans is uncommon. The flexures and neck typically show epidermal thickening and pigmentation (Fig. 1), and the skin is velvety or papillomatous. Warty lesions are seen around the mouth and on the palms and soles. *Pseudoacanthosis nigricans* describes similar changes seen with obesity or endocrine disorders such as acromegaly and insulin-resistant diabetes. Very rarely, acanthosis nigricans is *inherited* and appears in childhood or at puberty. The true condition, usually seen in a middle-aged or elderly subject, suggests a malignancy, most commonly of the gastrointestinal tract. Growth factors, released from the tumour or associated with the endocrine disorder, are thought to cause the skin changes. The underlying disease must be identified and treated.

ERYTHEMA GYRATUM REPENS

Erythema gyratum repens is an exceptionally rare pattern of concentric scaly rings of erythema which shift visibly from day-to-day (Fig. 2). The appearance resembles wood grain. An underlying neoplasm, frequently a carcinoma of the lung, is almost invariably found.

NECROLYTIC MIGRATORY ERYTHEMA

Necrolytic migratory erythema is a rare eruption of serpiginous erythematous plaques, with a migratory eroded edge. It typically starts in the perineum. The eruption indicates a tumour, or occasionally a hyperplasia, of the glucagon-secreting alpha cells of the pancreas (a *glucagonoma*). Weight loss, anaemia, mild diabetes, diarrhoea and glossitis are associated. Liver metastases are often present at diagnosis.

PAGET'S DISEASE AND EXTRA-MAMMARY PAGET'S DISEASE

Paget's disease presents as a unilateral eczema-like plaque of the nipple areola and represents the intraepidermal spread of an intraductal breast carcinoma. Extra-mammary Paget's disease is seen as an eczema-like eruption around the perineum or axilla. It usually results from intraepidermal spread of a ductal apocrine carcinoma. A skin biopsy confirms the diagnosis prior to surgical excision.

SECONDARY DEPOSITS

Cutaneous metastases are not uncommon. They occur late, indicate a poor prognosis, and may be the presenting sign of an internal tumour. Skin secondaries are multiple or solitary and appear as firm asymptomatic pink nodules (Fig. 3). The scalp, umbilicus and upper trunk are favoured sites. They occur most commonly with tumours of the breast, gastrointestinal tract, ovary and lung, and with malignant melanoma (p. 95). Leukaemias and lymphomas often show skin involvement (p. 98). Direct infiltration of the skin — carcinoma en cuirasse — is sometimes found with carcinoma of the breast (Fig. 4).

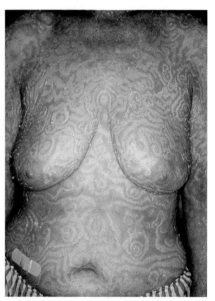
Fig. 2 **Erythema gyratum repens.** Note the 'wood grain' pattern.

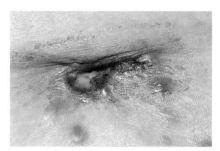
Fig. 3 **Secondary deposit at the umbilicus from a carcinoma of the breast.**

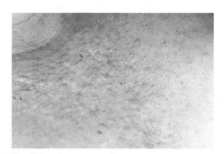
Fig. 4 **Carcinoma en cuirasse.** Direct pebbly infiltration of the skin of the chest wall from a carcinoma of the breast.

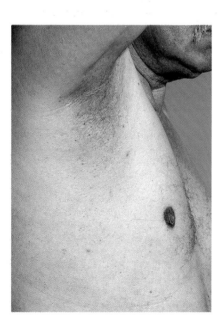
Fig. 1 **Acanthosis nigricans.** Pigmented velvety papillomatosis at the axilla and nipple are shown.

CONDITIONS OCCASIONALLY ASSOCIATED WITH MALIGNANCY

Conditions occasionally associated with underlying neoplasia but also seen with benign disease include:

- acquired ichthyosis
- dermatomyositis (p. 77)
- erythroderma (p. 40)
- flushing (p. 66)
- generalized pruritus
- hyperpigmentation
- hypertrichosis (p. 63)
- pyoderma gangrenosum
- superficial thrombophlebitis
- tylosis (p. 86).

ACQUIRED ICHTHYOSIS

Ichthyosis is usually inherited and starts in infancy (p. 86), but it may be acquired in adult life due to an underlying malignancy (e.g. Hodgkin's disease), essential fatty acid deficiency (e.g. caused by intestinal by-pass malabsorption), blood-lipid lowering drugs or leprosy therapy.

GENERALIZED PRURITUS

Generalized pruritus not associated with an eruption has several causes:

- idiopathic ('senile'): see page 110.
- iron deficiency
- liver disease
- malignancy, e.g. Hodgkin's disease
- neurological disorders
- polycythaemia
- renal failure
- thyroid dysfunction.

Patients with generalized pruritus need careful examination and investigation to exclude liver disease (e.g. biliary obstruction), iron deficiency, polycythaemia, hypothyroidism, hyperthyroidism and renal failure. Pruritus may occur with multiple sclerosis and neurofibromatosis. Sometimes, especially in the elderly, no cause is found and the itching is labelled *idiopathic*. The commonest malignant causes of pruritus are Hodgkin's disease (1/3 of patients with this itch) and polycythaemia rubra vera. The aetiology of the itching is poorly understood. Treatment, once any underlying disorder has been dealt with, is symptomatic. Sedative antihistamines, calamine lotion and topical antipruritics (e.g. 0.5% menthol or 1% phenol in aqueous cream) are used.

HYPERPIGMENTATION

Malignancy-associated pigmentation may result from ectopic ACTH or MSH-like hormone production by the tumour. It is also seen in patients with malignant cachexia. The axillae, groins and nipples are involved.

PYODERMA GANGRENOSUM

Pyoderma gangrenosum starts as a pustule or inflamed nodule which breaks down to produce an ulcer with an undermined purplish margin and a surrounding erythema (Fig. 5). The ulcer may extend rapidly. Lesions may be multiple. A bacterial gangrene (e.g. necrotizing fasciitis, p. 45) is sometimes misdiagnosed. Pyoderma gangrenosum often occurs on the trunk or lower limbs. An immune aetiology is suggested. The following diseases are associated:

- ulcerative colitis
- Crohn's disease
- rheumatoid arthritis
- Behçet's syndrome (p. 113)
- multiple myeloma and monoclonal gammopathy
- leukaemia (a bullous form is seen).

Treatment is with systemic steroids or cyclosporin. Cases associated with bowel disease can improve as this is controlled.

SUPERFICIAL THROMBOPHLEBITIS

Migratory superficial thrombophlebitis, mainly associated with carcinoma of the pancreas or lung, also occurs with Behçet's syndrome.

Table 1 Cutaneous manifestations of malignancy

Condition associated	Commonest malignancies
Almost always	
Acanthosis nigricans	Gastrointestinal tract
Erythema gyratum repens	Lung
Extra-mammary Paget's disease	Apocrine glands
Necrolytic migratory erythema	Pancreas (alpha cells)
Paget's disease of the nipple	Breast
Skin secondaries	Breast, gastrointestinal, ovary, lung
Occasionally	
Acquired ichthyosis	Lymphoma (Hodgkin's disease)
Dermatomyositis	Lung, breast, stomach
Erythroderma	T cell lymphoma
Flushing	Carcinoid syndrome
Generalized pruritus	Hodgkin's disease, polycythaemia rubra vera
Hyperpigmentation	Cachectic malignancy
Hypertrichosis	Various tumours
Pyoderma gangrenosum	Leukaemia, myeloma
Superficial thrombophlebitis	Pancreas, lung
Tylosis	Oesophagus

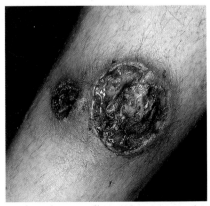

Fig. 5 **Pyoderma gangrenosum.** Necrotic ulcers shown here on the lower leg.

Associations with malignancy

- *Acanthosis nigricans*, characterized by pigmentation and epidermal thickening of the flexures, neck, palms and soles, is seen with gastrointestinal cancers.
- *Pseudoacanthosis nigricans* occurs with obesity or endocrine disorders.
- *Erythema gyratum repens* is a migratory erythema almost invariably associated with a neoplasm.
- *Paget's disease*, an eczema-like plaque at the nipple, is due to epidermal spread of an intraductal carcinoma. The *extra-mammary* form comes from an apocrine carcinoma.
- *Acquired ichthyosis* is associated with Hodgkin's disease, fatty acid deficiency and lipid-lowering drugs.
- *Generalized pruritus* may occur with malignancy (e.g. Hodgkin's disease), liver disease, renal failure, iron deficiency and thyroid dysfunction.
- *Pyoderma gangrenosum* is a necrotic ulceration seen with ulcerative colitis, Crohn's disease, rheumatoid arthritis, myeloma or leukaemia.

KERATINIZATION AND BLISTERING SYNDROMES

Common skin disorders, e.g. atopic eczema or psoriasis, have a genetic component that is often subject to environmental influences. The *genodermatoses* differ in being single gene defects and include keratinization, blistering and neurocutaneous syndromes.

THE ICHTHYOSES

The ichthyoses are inherited disorders of keratinization and epidermal differentiation. They are characterized by dry scaly skin and vary from mild and asymptomatic to severe and incompatible with life (Table 1). Keratinization is abnormal. Some of the biochemical defects have been identified, e.g. steroid sulphatase is deficient in sex-linked ichthyosis.

Clinical presentation

Ichthyosis vulgaris is common and unrecognized if mild. Small branny scales are seen on the extensor aspects of the limbs and the back (Fig. 1). The flexures are often spared.

The other types of ichthyosis are uncommon or rare and can usually be identified by their clinical features, onset and inheritance. Autosomal dominant conditions tend to improve with age, whereas recessive ichthyoses may worsen. *Collodion baby* describes a newborn infant with a tight shiny skin which causes feeding problems and ectropion. It is mainly due to non-bullous ichthyosiform erythroderma. *Acquired ichthyosis* (p. 85) usually starts in adulthood.

Table 1 **A classification of the ichthyoses**

Disorder	Inheritance	Clinical features
Ichthyosis vulgaris	Autosomal-dominant	Common (1 in 300). Onset 1–4 year. It occurs with atopy. Often mild. Small bran-like scale seen. Flexures spared
Sex-linked ichthyosis	X-linked-recessive	1 in 2000 males. Generalized involvement with large brown scale. Onset in first week of life. Improves in summer. Due to a deficiency of steroid sulphatase
Non-bullous ichthyosiform erythroderma*	Autosomal-recessive	Rare. At birth may present as collodion baby. Red scaly skin and ectropion may follow. Erythema improves with age
Bullous ichthyosiform erythroderma**	Autosomal-dominant	Rare. Redness and blisters occur after birth but fade. Warty rippled hyperkeratosis appears in childhood

* Lamellar ichthyosis is similar but rarer ** Also called epidermolytic hyperkeratosis

Management

Emollient ointments, creams and bath additives (p. 20) are essential, and adequate for mild ichthyosis. Urea-containing creams (e.g. Aquadrate or Calmurid) help, but severe forms may need acitretin (p. 29).

KERATODERMA

Keratoderma describes gross hyperkeratosis of the palms and soles, and may be acquired or inherited.

Clinical presentation

The degrees of involvement and modes of inheritance vary. A common pattern, *tylosis*, shows diffuse hyperkeratosis of the palms and soles (Fig. 2) and is usually of autosomal-dominant inheritance. In a few families, tylosis is associated with carcinoma of the oesophagus. Other keratodermas may give punctate papular lesions on the palms and soles or, in 'mutilating' types, fibrous bands that strangulate digits.

Acquired palmo-plantar keratoderma is seen in pityriasis rubra pilaris (p. 40) and lichen planus and may develop in women at the menopause, particularly around the heels. Corns and callosities are different from keratoderma. *Callosities* are painless localized thickenings of the keratin layer and are seen as a protective response, induced by friction or pressure, that is often occupational in origin. *Corns* are painful and develop at areas of high local pressure on the feet, where shoes squeeze against bony points.

Management

Treatment is with keratolytics, e.g. 5–10% salicylic acid ointment or 10% urea cream. Sometimes the use of acitretin is justified.

KERATOSIS PILARIS

Keratosis pilaris is a common, sometimes inherited condition in which multiple small horny follicular plugs affect the upper thigh, upper arm and face (Fig. 3). It is sometimes associated with ichthyosis vulgaris. Application of 5% salicylic acid ointment or 10% urea cream lessens but does not cure the problem.

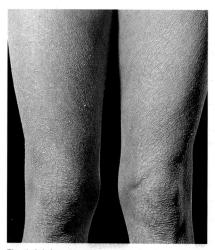

Fig. 1 **Ichthyosis vulgaris showing bran-like scaling.**

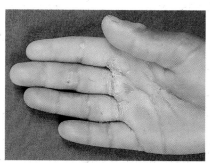

Fig. 2 **Keratoderma of the palm.**

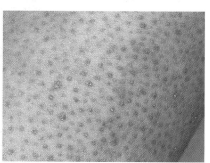

Fig. 3 **Keratosis pilaris on the upper arm.**

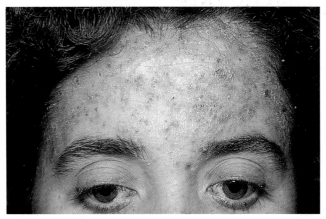

Fig. 4 **Darier's disease affecting the forehead.**

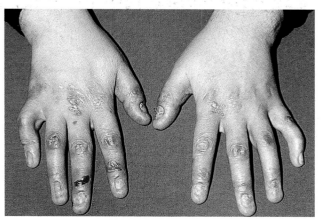

Fig. 5 **Epidermolysis bullosa.** The dystrophic-dominant type is shown.

DARIER'S DISEASE

Darier's disease (keratosis follicularis) is a rare autosomal-dominant condition characterized by brownish scaly papules. The abnormal gene is sited on chromosome 12. Keratinocyte tonofilaments and desmosomes are defective on electron microscopy and a keratin anomaly is likely.

Clinical presentation

The disease presents in teenagers or young adults, with small brown greasy-scaled papules, typically on the flexures, upper back, chest and forehead (Fig. 4). Its onset may follow sunburn. The severity varies from being mild and almost unnoticed to being extensive and severe. Nail changes (p. 64) and palmar pits or keratoses are found. Eczema herpeticum (p. 33) may occur.

Management

Mild Darier's disease requires topical keratolytics only (e.g. 5% salicylic acid ointment). More severe cases are helped greatly by acitretin (p. 29).

FLEGEL'S DISEASE

Flegel's disease (hyperkeratosis lenticularis perstans) is a rare, dominantly inherited disorder, characterized by keratotic plugs on the legs and arms. It starts in middle age. When larger plugs are seen it is called *Kyrle's disease*, but the two types may coexist.

EPIDERMOLYSIS BULLOSA

Epidermolysis bullosa (EB) defines a group of genetically inherited diseases characterized by blistering on minimal trauma. They range from being mild and trivial to being incompatible with life (Table 2).

Aetiopathogenesis

Keratin synthesis is defective in simple EB (genes mapped to chromosomes 12 and 17). Collagen VII is abnormal in dystrophic EB (gene sited on chromosome 3). Anchoring fibrils (p. 2) are defective in certain types of *EB*.

Clinical presentation and management

Simple EB is fairly common and requires avoidance of trauma. The more severe forms (Table 2; Fig. 5) need to be managed in specialized centres. Avoidance of trauma, supportive measures and the control of infection are important. Treatment with various drugs has given disappointing results. *Acquired EB*, with an onset in adult life, shows trauma-induced blistering and resembles pemphigoid on immunofluorescent studies.

PRENATAL DIAGNOSIS OF INHERITED DISORDERS

DNA-based prenatal diagnosis is now possible for junctional and recessive dystrophic EB, bullous ichthyosiform erythroderma, and oculocutaneous albinism. DNA is obtained from chorionic villus samples or amniotic cells. Fetal skin biopsy, done at 16–24 weeks, remains the only way to detect non-bullous ichthyosiform erythroderma.

Table 2 **The main types of epidermolysis bullosa**

Disease	Inheritance	Clinical features
Simple EB	Autosomal-dominant	Commonest type. Often mild and limited to hands and feet. Blisters caused by friction. Nails and mouth unaffected
Junctional EB	Autosomal-recessive	Rare and often lethal. At birth large erosions seen around mouth and anus. Slow to heal. No effective treatment
Dystrophic EB	Autosomal-dominant	Hands, knees and elbows are affected. Scarring with milia is found. Deformity of the nails may occur
Dystrophic EB	Autosomal-recessive	Starts in infancy. Severe blistering results in fusion of fingers and toes, with mucosal lesions and oesophageal stricture

Inherited keratinization and blistering disorders

- *The ichthyoses* are inherited disorders of keratinization. The skin is dry and scaly. Certain ichthyoses may present at birth as a collodion baby.
- *Darier's disease* is a rare autosomal-dominant condition. Greasy scaly papules are seen on the chest, back and in the flexures. Severe cases are treated with retinoids.
- *Keratoderma* is typified by hyperkeratosis of the palms and soles and is treated by keratolytics.
- *Keratosis pilaris* is a common condition in which horny follicular plugs are seen on the limbs and face.
- *Epidermolysis bullosa* describes inherited bullous diseases ranging from mild blistering induced by ill-fitting shoes to severe and lethal blistering present at birth.

NEUROCUTANEOUS DISORDERS AND OTHER SYNDROMES

Certain inherited skin disorders also have significant involvement of internal organs. The neurocutaneous disorders, the inherited diseases of connective tissue and the premature ageing syndromes are included.

NEUROFIBROMATOSIS

Von Recklinghausen's neurofibromatosis (NF1) is relatively common, affecting about 1 in 5000 of the population. It is characterized by café-au-lait spots, cutaneous neurofibromas and other bony or neurological abnormalities. The disease shows autosomal-dominant inheritance, although 50% of cases are new mutations.

Aetiopathogenesis

The NF1 gene has been mapped to chromosome 17. This finding offers the prospect of devising a prenatal DNA screening test to identify those at risk.

Clinical presentation

The two main cutaneous features are:

- *Café-au-lait spots*: round or oval coffee-coloured macules, due to increased melanin pigment. They often appear in the first year of life. One or two café-au-lait spots are seen in 10% of normal people but, in neurofibromatosis, six or more are usually present. Freckling of the axilla is also found (Fig. 1).
- *Dermal neurofibromas*: small nodules which appear around the time of puberty and increase in number throughout life (Fig. 2). Their number varies from a few to several hundred.

A proportion of patients with NF1 have short stature and macrocephaly. Rare variants of the disease are occasionally seen. The commonest is NF2 (*central neurofibromatosis*) in which patients have bilateral acoustic neuromas but few if any café-au-lait spots or dermal nodules. NF2 also shows autosomal-dominant inheritance. The NF2 gene is on chromosome 22.

Complications

Complications develop in about 25% of cases and include the following:

- *Plexiform neurofibromas* are larger than their dermal counterparts and measure up to several cm in size. They are associated with

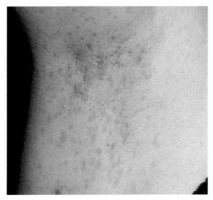

Fig. 1 **Neurofibromatosis showing axillary freckling.**

pigmentation and hypertrophy of the overlying skin or underlying bone, and present a cosmetic problem.
- *Benign tumours of the nervous system* may develop. These include optic gliomas, acoustic neuromas and spinal neurofibromas which arise from nerve roots of the spinal cord.
- *Sarcomatous change* in a neurofibroma occurs in 1.5–15% of cases.
- *Scoliosis* or bowing of the tibia and fibula may occur.
- *Other problems* include hypertension, epilepsy and learning difficulties.

Management

Once the diagnosis has been made, genetic counselling and the exclusion of any complicating factors are important. Troublesome nodules can be excised, and larger disfiguring neurofibromas removed by plastic surgery. Patients are often helped by a patient support group (p. 120).

TUBEROUS SCLEROSIS

Tuberous sclerosis is an uncommon autosomal-dominant condition of variable expression. About 50% of patients are new mutations. Hamartomas occur in several organs. The abnormal genes have been mapped to chromosomes 9 and 11.

Clinical manifestations

The features may not appear until puberty. Patients typically show:

- *Adenoma sebaceum*: red or yellow fibromatous papules that are usually found around the nose (Fig. 3).
- *Periungual fibromas*: pink fibrous projections are seen under the nailfolds (Fig. 4).

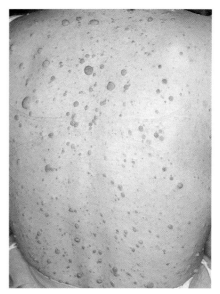

Fig. 2 **Neurofibromatosis.** Multiple neurofibromas are present on the back.

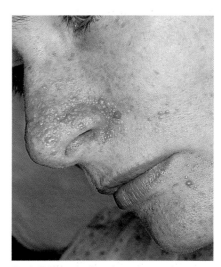

Fig. 3 **Tuberous sclerosis.** 'Adenoma sebaceum' are seen at the sides of the nose.

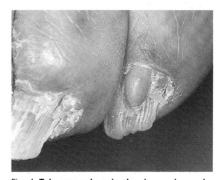

Fig. 4 **Tuberous sclerosis showing periungual fibromas.**

- *Shagreen patches*: connective tissue naevi, yellowish with a cobblestone surface, are found on the back.

- *Ash-leaf macules*: small white oval macules, sometimes present at birth, and best seen with a Wood's light.
- *Neurological involvement*: mental retardation and epilepsy are common. Intracranial calcification is seen.
- *Other features*: retinal gliomas, cardiac rhabdomyomas and renal tumours are found.

Management

An affected individual should have a full clinical examination, often with radiographs and CT scan of the head. Children are screened for ash-leaf macules using a Wood's light. The adenoma sebaceum may be improved by hyfrecation or laser, but tend to recur. Genetic counselling is given once the diagnosis is made. The support group is helpful (p. 120).

INCONTINENTIA PIGMENTI

Incontinentia pigmenti is a rare X-linked-dominant condition which is usually lethal *in utero* in males. In females it presents within a few days of birth as a widespread blistering eruption (p. 13). Warty papules follow, but are replaced by hyperpigmentation which appears in a whorled pattern. Skeletal, ocular, neurological and dental abnormalities are associated.

XERODERMA PIGMENTOSUM

Xeroderma pigmentosum is a group of rare autosomal-recessive conditions, characterized by defective repair of ultraviolet-damaged DNA. Photosensitivity begins in infancy, and freckles and keratoses appear on exposed skin in childhood. Squamous cell and basal cell carcinomas, keratoacanthomas and malignant melanomas subsequently develop in the UV-damaged skin (Fig. 5). Strict sunlight avoidance is necessary, but in its severe form the disease is fatal in the second or third decade. The gene loci are known (p. 12). Prenatal diagnosis is possible (p. 87) and is used when parents have already had one affected child.

EHLERS-DANLOS SYNDROME

More than 10 inherited disorders of defective collagen structure and biochemistry are included in this group of conditions (gene loci: p. 12). The diseases may be dominant, recessive or X-linked, and present in varying degrees of severity. The features include:
- elasticity of the skin
- joint hyperextensibility
- skin fragility with bruising and scarring (Fig. 6).

In the more severe types, aneurysms and rupture of large arteries may be found.

PSEUDOXANTHOMA ELASTICUM

Pseudoxanthoma elasticum describes a group of at least four disorders, characterized by abnormalities in elastin and, probably, collagen. The inheritance is autosomal-recessive or dominant. The skin is loose, wrinkled and yellow, and contains small papules (resembling xanthomas) giving a 'chicken skin' appearance. These changes are most obvious at the neck and flexures. Angioid streaks in the retina are seen in more than 50% of cases. Arterial involvement may result in gastrointestinal or cerebral haemorrhage.

THE PREMATURE AGEING SYNDROMES

The features of ageing include an increased susceptibility to neoplasia, dementia, diabetes, autoimmune disease, cataracts, premature alopecia and hair greying, osteoporosis and degenerative vascular disease. *Down's syndrome* shows several of these stigmata and is the most common condition in which premature ageing occurs. Many of the other disorders of premature ageing, such as *Werner's syndrome* or *progeria*, are very rare and often of autosomal-recessive inheritance.

Aged skin is dry, wrinkled, atrophic, shows loss of elasticity and uneven pigmentation, and is susceptible to develop benign and malignant tumours. Photoageing from chronic sun exposure (p. 100) can produce similar changes, although certain of the features are more prominent. Some conditions, such as pseudoxanthoma elasticum or xeroderma pigmentosum, have the signs of aged skin without necessarily showing more generalized features of ageing.

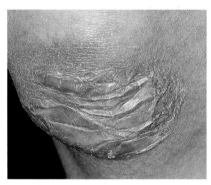

Fig. 6 **Ehlers-Danlos syndrome.** Ugly scarring has resulted from fragile skin and poor wound healing.

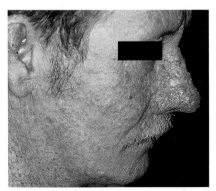

Fig. 5 **Xeroderma pigmentosum.** This patient shows severely sun-damaged skin with freckling, keratoses and scars from excision of tumours.

Neurocutaneous disorders and other syndromes

- *NF1 neurofibromatosis* is a relatively common autosomal-dominant condition characterized by café-au-lait spots, dermal neurofibromas and sometimes skeletal or neurological anomalies. The abnormal gene is on chromosome 17.
- *Tuberous sclerosis* is an uncommon autosomal-dominant disorder with prominent skin signs (e.g. adenoma sebaceum and periungual fibromas), mental retardation and epilepsy.
- *Incontinentia pigmenti* is a rare X-linked-dominant disease, present at birth, which evolves through vesicular and warty stages to leave whorled patterns of pigmentation.
- *Xeroderma pigmentosum* represents a group of rare recessive conditions showing defects of DNA repair, characterized by skin tumours and premature death.
- *Ehlers-Danlos syndrome* is a group of inherited collagen disorders in which skin elasticity and joint hypermobility are found.
- *Pseudoxanthoma elasticum* represents diseases of defective elastin. The skin is wrinkled with yellowish papules. Retinal changes are seen.

BENIGN TUMOURS

Skin tumours are common, and their incidence is rising in Western countries (p. 22). The treatment of skin tumours makes up a large part of current dermatological practice (p. 22). Many skin tumours are benign, and these are described in this section. Viral warts, actinic keratoses and naevi are mentioned elsewhere.

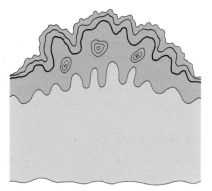

Fig. 1 **Histopathology of a seborrhoeic wart.** The illustration shows a hyperkeratotic epidermis, thickened by basal cell proliferation, with keratin cysts.

BENIGN EPIDERMAL TUMOURS

SEBORRHOEIC WART (BASAL CELL PAPILLOMA)

A seborrhoeic wart (seborrhoeic keratosis) is a common, usually pigmented, benign tumour consisting of a proliferation of basal keratinocytes (Fig. 1). The cause is unknown. Seborrhoea is not associated.

Clinical presentation
Seborrhoeic warts have the following features:

- often multiple (Fig. 2), sometimes solitary
- affect the elderly or middle-aged
- mostly found on the trunk and face
- generally round or oval in shape
- start as small papules, often lightly pigmented or yellow
- become darkly pigmented warty nodules 1–6 cm in diameter
- have a 'stuck-on' appearance, with keratin plugs and well-defined edges.

Differential diagnosis
The diagnosis is usually obvious from the physical findings and multiplicity of the lesions. Occasionally, a seborrhoeic wart can resemble an actinic keratosis, melanocytic naevus, pigmented basal cell carcinoma or malignant melanoma.

Management
Multiple lesions can be adequately dealt with using liquid nitrogen cryotherapy. Thicker seborrhoeic warts are best treated by curettage or shave biopsy, with cautery or hyfrecation. If there is doubt about the diagnosis, excision and histological examination are advised.

SKIN TAGS

Skin tags are pedunculated benign fibroepithelial polyps, a few mm in length. They are common, mainly seen in the elderly or middle-aged, and show a predilection for the neck, axillae, groin and eyelids (Fig. 3). The cause is unknown, but they are often found in obese individuals. Occasionally, skin tags are confused with small melanocytic naevi or seborrhoeic warts. The treatment, usually for cos-

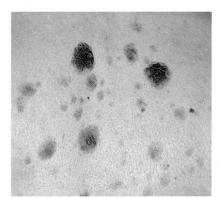

Fig. 2 **Seborrhoeic warts on the trunk, with a few small Campbell-de-Morgan spots.**

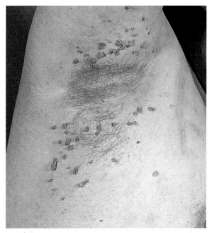

Fig. 3 **Skin tags in the axilla.**

metic reasons, is by snipping the stalk with scissors or cutting through it with a hyfrecator (under local anaesthetic if necessary), or by using cryotherapy.

EPIDERMAL CYST

Epidermal cysts, usually seen on the scalp, face or trunk, are sometimes incorrectly called sebaceous cysts. They are keratin-filled and derived from the epidermis or, in the case of the related pilar cyst, the outer root sheath of the hair follicle. The cysts are firm, skin coloured, mobile and normally 1–3 cm in diameter. Bacterial infection is a complication. Excision is curative.

MILIUM

Milia are mostly seen on the face, where they typically appear as small white keratin cysts (1–2 mm in size) around the eyelids and on the upper cheeks. They are often seen in children but may appear at any age. Occasionally, milia may develop as part of healing after a subepidermal blister, e.g. with porphyria cutanea tarda. Milial cysts can normally be extracted using a sterile needle.

BENIGN DERMAL TUMOURS

DERMATOFIBROMA (HISTIOCYTOMA)

Dermatofibromas are common dermal nodules, and are usually asymptomatic. Histologically, they show a proliferation of fibroblasts, with dermal fibrosis and sometimes epidermal hyperplasia. They may represent a reaction pattern to an insect bite or other trauma, although often no such history is obtained.

Clinical presentation
Dermatofibromas are usually seen in young adults, most commonly women, and mainly occur on the lower legs.

They are firm, dermal nodules 5–10mm in diameter and may be pigmented (Fig. 4). They enlarge slowly, if at all.

Management

A pigmented dermatofibroma may be confused with a melanocytic naevus or a malignant melanoma. Excision of symptomatic or diagnostically doubtful lesions is recommended.

PYOGENIC GRANULOMA

A pyogenic granuloma is a rapidly developing bright red or blood-crusted nodule which may be confused with a malignant melanoma. It is neither pyogenic nor granulomatous but is an acquired haemangioma.

Clinical presentation

A pyogenic granuloma typically:

- develops at a site of trauma, e.g. a prick from a thorn
- presents as a bright red, sometimes pedunculated, nodule which bleeds easily (Fig. 5)
- enlarges rapidly over 2–3 weeks
- is seen on a finger (also on lip, face and foot)
- occurs in young adults or children.

Management

Curettage and cautery, or excision, is needed. The specimen is sent for histological examination to exclude a malignant melanoma. Not infrequently, a pyogenic granuloma may recur after curettage.

KELOID

A keloid is an excessive proliferation of connective tissue in response to skin trauma and differs from a hypertrophic scar because it extends beyond the limit of the original injury. Keloids show the following characteristics:

- present as protuberant and firm smooth nodules or plaques (Fig. 6)
- occur mainly over the upper back, chest and ear lobes
- develop more commonly in Black Africans
- have their highest incidence in the second to fourth decades.

Treatment is by the injection of steroid into the keloid.

CAMPBELL-DE-MORGAN SPOT (CHERRY ANGIOMA)

Campbell-de-Morgan spots are benign capillary proliferations, commonly seen as small bright-red papules on the trunk in elderly or

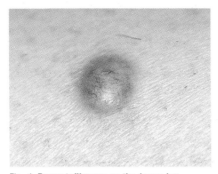
Fig. 4 **Dermatofibroma on the lower leg.**

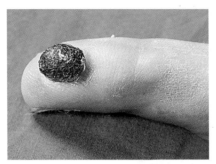
Fig. 5 **Pyogenic granuloma on the finger.**

middle-aged patients (see Fig. 2). If necessary they can be removed by hyfrecation or cautery.

LIPOMA

Lipomas are benign tumours of fat, and present as soft masses in the subcutaneous tissue. They are often multiple and are mostly found on the trunk, neck and upper extremities. Sometimes they are painful. Removal is rarely needed.

CHONDRODERMATITIS NODULARIS

Chondrodermatitis nodularis is not a neoplasm but presents as a small painful nodule on the upper rim of the helix of the pinna, usually in elderly men. It is due to inflammation in the cartilage which may be a response to degenerative changes in the dermis. They are often confused with basal cell carcinomas. Excision is curative.

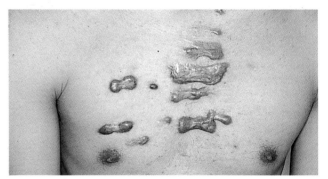
Fig. 6 **Keloids.** The nodules are seen on the chest of a patient with a history of acne.

Benign tumours

Lesion	Age at onset	Main features
Epidermal		
Viral wart	Childhood mainly	Usually on hands or feet (p. 48)
Actinic keratosis	Old age	Sun-exposed areas (p. 101)
Seborrhoeic wart	Old/middle age	Keratosis, often on trunk
Milia	Childhood	White cysts, often on the face
Epidermal cyst	After childhood	Most on face or scalp
Skin tags	Middle/old age	Seen on neck and axillae
Dermal		
Dermatofibroma	Young adult, F > M	Nodule, often on leg
Melanocytic naevus	Teens/young adult	Brown macule or papule (p. 92)
Cherry angioma	Old/middle age	Small red papule on trunk
Pyogenic granuloma	Child/young adult	Red nodule, often on finger
Keloid	2nd–4th decades	Chest and neck, often in negroids
Lipoma	Any age	Soft tumour on trunk or limbs
Chondrodermatitis nodularis	Old/middle age	Nodule on pinna, M > F

NAEVI

A naevus is a benign proliferation of one or more of the normal constituent cells of the skin. Naevi may be present at birth or may develop later. The commonest naevi are those containing benign collections of melanocytic naevus cells, but other types of naevi are found (Table 1).

MELANOCYTIC NAEVI

Melanocytic naevi ('moles') are common. They are present in most caucasoids but are less prevalent in mongoloids and Black Africans.

Aetiopathogenesis and pathology

The naevus cells in melanocytic naevi are thought to be derived from melanocytes which migrate to the epidermis from the neural crest during embryonic development (p. 2). The reason for the development of naevi is unknown, but they seem to be an inherited trait in many families.

The position of the naevus cells within the dermis determines the type of naevus (Fig. 1). The junctional type has clusters of naevus cells at the dermo-epidermal junction, the intradermal type has nests of naevus cells in the dermis, and the compound naevus shows both components.

Naevus cells produce melanin, and if the pigment is deep in the dermis, an optical effect can give the lesion a blue colour, as in a blue naevus.

Clinical presentation

A congenital naevus, that is one present at birth, is seen in about 1% of caucasoids, but most naevi develop during childhood or adolescence. Their number reaches a peak at puberty, and they tend to become less numerous during adult life. However, it is not unusual to see a few new naevi appear during the third decade, especially if provoked by excessive sun exposure or pregnancy. The average caucasoid has between 10 and 30 or more melanocytic naevi. The clinical features are as follows:

- *Congenital naevi.* Present at birth, they are usually more than 1 cm in size, vary in colour from light brown to black, and often become protuberant and hairy. They can be disfiguring, as in the rare bathing trunk naevus, and carry a risk (perhaps up to 5%) for the development of malignant melanoma (p. 95).
- *Junctional naevi.* These are flat macules, varying in size from 2–10 mm and in colour from light to dark brown (Fig. 2). They are usually round or oval in shape and have a predilection for the palms, soles and genitalia.
- *Intradermal naevi.* The intradermal naevus is a dome-shaped papule or nodule which may be skin coloured or pigmented, and is most often seen on the face or neck.
- *Compound naevi.* Compound naevi are usually less than 10 mm in diameter, have a smooth surface and vary in their degree of pigmentation (Fig. 3). Larger lesions may develop a warty or cerebriform appearance. They may occur anywhere on the skin surface.
- *Spitz naevi.* A spitz neavus is a firm, reddish-brown, rounded nodule seen typically on the face of a child. The initial growth may be rapid. Histologically, the naevas cells are proliferative and the dermal vessels are dilated.
- *Blue naevi.* This variant, so-called because of its steely-blue colour, is usually solitary and is most common on the extremities, particularly the hands and feet.
- *Halo naevi.* Halo (or Sutton's) naevi are mainly seen on the trunk in children or adolescents and represent the destruction, by the body's immune system, of

Table 1 **A classification of naevi**

Group	Example
Melanocytic	Congenital (p. 95)
	Junctional
	Intradermal
	Compound
	Spitz
	Blue
	Halo
	Becker's
	Dysplastic (p. 95)
Vascular	Salmon patch (p. 109)
	Port wine stain (p. 109)
	Strawberry (p. 109)
	Cavernous haemangioma
Epidermal	Warty naevus
Connective tissue	Tuberous sclerosis (p. 88)

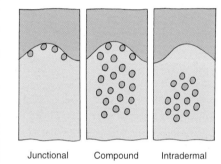

Junctional   Compound   Intradermal

Fig. 1 **Types of melanocytic naevi.** The site of the naevus cells, either at the dermo-epidermal junction or in the dermis, or at both places, determines the type of melanocytic naevus.

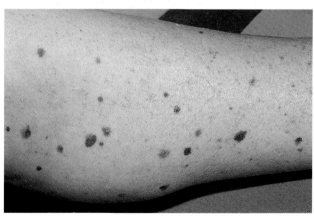

Fig. 2 **Multiple junctional (and compound) naevi on the lower leg.**

naevus cells in a naevus. A white halo of depigmentation surrounds the pre-existing naevus which subsequently involutes (Fig. 4). The reason for this is not known, but there is an association with vitiligo. Multiple halos often appear simultaneously.
- *Becker's naevi.* This rare variant usually develops in adolescent males as a unilateral lesion on the upper back or chest (Fig. 5). Hyperpigmented at first, it later becomes hairy.
- *Dysplastic naevi.* See page 95.

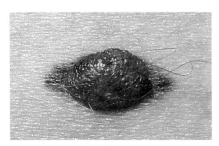

Fig. 3 **Compound melanocytic naevus.**

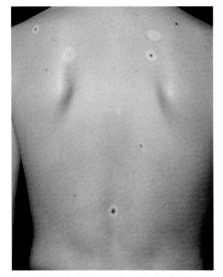

Fig. 4 **Multiple halo naevi on the back of an adolescent.**

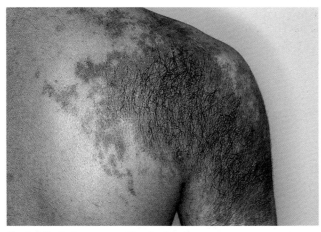

Fig. 5 **A Becker's naevus on the shoulder in a young man.**

Management

Over recent years, publicity in the media and public health campaigns have promoted the early diagnosis of malignant melanoma. This has lead to a greater public awareness about the significance of change in pigmented lesions, and many patients are now referred because of concern about their 'moles'. Any change merits serious attention (p. 95). The differential diagnosis of melanocytic naevi is shown in Table 2. Naevi are excised because of:

- *concern about malignancy*, e.g. recent increase in size or itching
- *an increased risk of malignant change*, e.g. in a large congenital naevus
- *cosmetic reasons*, e.g. ugly naevi, usually on the face or neck
- *repeated inflammation*, e.g. bacterial folliculitis
- *recurrent trauma*, e.g. naevi on the back which catch on bra straps.

All excised naevi should be sent for histology. Some clearly benign protuberant naevi, being removed for cosmetic reasons, can be dealt with by shave biopsy (p. 105).

EPIDERMAL NAEVI

Epidermal naevi usually are present at birth or develop in early childhood. They are warty, often pigmented, and frequently linear (Fig. 6). Most are a few cm long, but they can be much larger and involve the length of a limb or the side of the trunk. They can be excised, but recurrence is common. A variant on the scalp, *naevus sebaceous*, carries a risk of malignant transformation and should be excised.

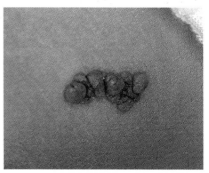

Fig. 6 **An epidermal naevus on the thigh.**

CONNECTIVE TISSUE NAEVI

Connective tissue naevi are rare. They appear as smooth, skin-coloured papules or plaques and may be multiple. Coarse collagen bundles are seen in the dermis on histology. An example is the cobblestone naevus (shagreen patch) seen in tuberous sclerosis (p. 88).

Table 2 **Differential diagnosis of melanocytic naevi**

Lesion	Distinguishing features
Freckle	Tan-coloured macules on sun-exposed sites (p. 71)
Lentigine	Usually multiple, onset in later life (p. 71)
Seborrhoeic wart	Stuck-on appearance, warty lesions, may show keratin plugs, but easily confused (p. 90)
Haemangioma	Vascular but may show pigmentation
Dermatofibroma	On legs, elevated nodule, firm and pigmented (p. 90)
Pigmented basal cell carcinoma	Often on face, pearly edge, increase in size, can ulcerate, other photodamage may co-exist
Malignant melanoma	Variable colour and outline, increase in size, may be inflamed or itchy (p. 94)

Naevi

- **Melanocytic naevi** are very common, usually multiple, pigmented and benign. They appear during childhood or adolescence. Variants include:
  - *Congenital naevi* are present at birth, may be protuberant or hairy, and have a small risk of malignant change.
  - *Junctional naevi* are flat macules, often round or oval-shaped. Typically found on soles, palms or genitalia.
  - *Intradermal naevi* are dome-shaped, usually skin-coloured papules. Typically seen on the face.
  - *Compound naevi* are pigmented nodules or papules, sometimes warty or hairy.
  - *Blue naevi* are steely-blue in colour, mainly solitary, and found on the extremities.
  - *Halo naevi* show depigmentation where a naevus has involuted. Mostly seen on the trunk.
- **Epidermal naevi** are warty, pigmented and often linear. Usually small, they are sometimes extensive.
- **Connective tissue naevi** are skin-coloured papules composed of coarse collagen in the dermis.

MALIGNANT MELANOMA

Malignant melanoma is a malignant tumour of melanocytes, usually arising in the epidermis. It is the most lethal of the main skin tumours and has increased in incidence over the last few years. Malignant melanoma has received attention from public education campaigns, particularly because of its putative relationship to episodes of excessive ultraviolet radiation exposure.

CLINICAL PRESENTATION

Four main clinico-pathological variants are recognized. These are described below.

Superficial spreading malignant melanoma

This type accounts for 50% of all UK cases, shows a female preponderance, and is commonest on the lower leg. The tumour is macular and shows variable pigmentation often with regression (Fig. 1).

Lentigo malignant melanoma

Malignant melanoma developing in a long-standing lentigo maligna (Fig. 3) comprises 15% of UK cases. A lentigo maligna arises in sun-damaged skin often on the face of an elderly person who has spent many years in an outdoor occupation.

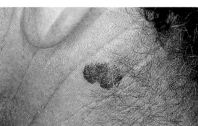

Fig. 1 **Superficial spreading malignant melanoma.**

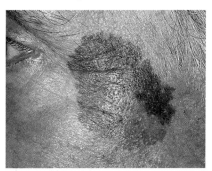

Fig. 3 **Lentigo maligna** showing irregular outline and pigmentation.

Acral lentiginous malignant melanoma

The acral-lentiginous type makes up only 10% of UK cases but is the commonest form in mongoloids. The tumour affects the palms, soles (Fig. 4) and nail beds, is often diagnosed late, and has poor survival figures.

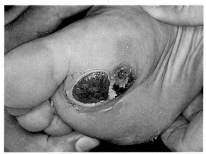

Fig. 4 **Acral lentiginous malignant melanoma.**

Nodular malignant melanoma

The nodular variant is seen in 25% of British patients, shows a male preponderance, and is commonest on the trunk. The pigmented nodule (Fig. 2) may grow rapidly and ulcerate.

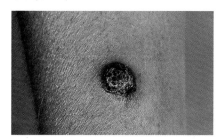

Fig. 2 **Nodular malignant melanoma.**

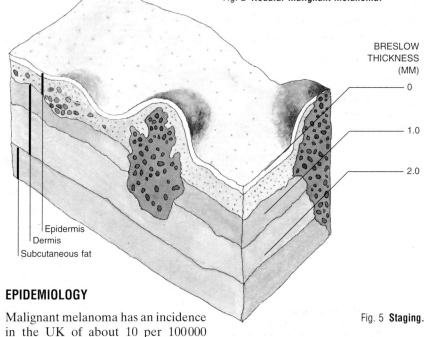

BRESLOW THICKNESS (MM)

0

1.0

2.0

Epidermis
Dermis
Subcutaneous fat

Fig. 5 **Staging.**

EPIDEMIOLOGY

Malignant melanoma has an incidence in the UK of about 10 per 100 000 population per year. The incidence is rising 7% yearly and doubling every decade. It occurs in all races but is particularly a problem in caucasoids, in whom it becomes much more common the closer the population lives to the equator. In the UK, women are affected twice as frequently as men. Superficial spreading and nodular melanomas tend to occur in those in the 20–60 year age group, while lentigo malignant melanomas mostly affect those over 60 years old. In males, the commonest site is the back; in females, it is the lower leg (about half occur here).

STAGING

Malignant melanomas usually though not invariably progress through two stages (Fig. 5), horizontal and vertical. The *horizontal* phase of malignant melanocytic growth within the epidermis may evolve into a stage of dermal involvement and *vertical* growth.

Local invasion by the tumour is assessed using the *Breslow method*, which is the measurement in mm of the distance between the granular cell layer to the deepest identifiable melanoma cell. Metastasis is uncommon in tumours restricted to the epidermis.

AETIOPATHOGENESIS

The cause of malignant melanoma is not known, but repeated short, intensive, exposure to ultraviolet radiation, e.g. on sun-seeking holidays, may be involved. Major risk factors are shown in Figure 6. Histological evidence of a pre-existing melanocytic naevus is found in 30% of malignant melanomas but, with the exception of dysplastic or congenital naevi (Fig. 7), the risk of change in a common melanocytic naevus is small.

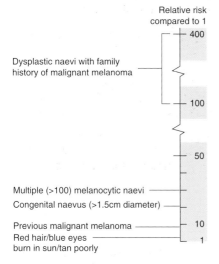

Fig. 6 **Major risk factors.** The major risk factors and their relative risk for the development of malignant melanoma are shown.

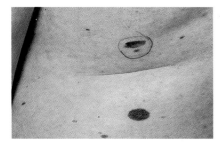

Fig. 7 **Dysplastic naevus syndrome.** This condition, which may be familial, is characterized by large numbers of atypical and 'dysplastic' naevi, which are often over 7mm in diameter with an irregular edge and variable pigmentation. Affected individuals have a greatly increased risk of developing malignant melanoma. They should avoid the sun and be closely observed. Changing or suspicious pigmented lesions should be excised for histological examination.

DIAGNOSIS

Any of the following changes in a naevus or pigmented lesion may suggest malignant melanoma:

- *size* : usually a recent increase
- *shape* : irregular in outline
- *colour*: variation
- *inflammation*: may be at the edge
- *crusting*: some ooze or bleed
- *itch*: a common symptom.

The *differential diagnosis* of malignant melanoma includes:

- benign melanocytic naevus (p. 92)
- seborrhoeic wart (p. 90)
- haemangioma (p. 91)
- dermatofibroma (p. 90)
- pigmented basal cell carcinoma (p. 96)
- benign lentigo (p. 71).

PROGNOSIS

The prognosis relates to the tumour depth. Tumours are usually divided into three prognosis groups: good (thickness less than 1.5mm), intermediate (1.5–3.5mm) and poor (>3.5mm). The approximate 5-year survival rates for these groups are:

- <1.49mm   93%
- 1.5–3.49mm   67%
- >3.5mm   38%

Examples of thin and thick tumours are given in Figures 8 and 9.

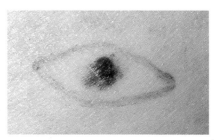

Fig. 8 **A thin (0.8 mm Breslow thickness) superficial spreading malignant melanoma with a good prognosis.**

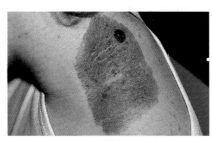

Fig. 9 **A thick (11 mm Breslow thickness) nodular malignant melanoma developing within a large congenital naevus.** Local lymph nodes were involved and the prognosis was poor.

MANAGEMENT

The primary treatment is surgical excision. Tumours of a thickness of 1mm or less require a 1cm clearance margin. Tumours of more than 1.0mm in thickness need a 2–3cm clearance, and often a skin graft is necessary to close the defect. Regular follow-up is needed to detect any recurrence. Three main types recur:

- *local* (Fig. 10)
- *lymphatic* — either in the regional lymph nodes or in transit in the lymphatics draining from the tumour to the nodes
- *blood-borne* to distant sites.

Prophylactic excision of local lymph nodes is used in some centres for intermediate or thick tumours. Radiotherapy is of limited use. Clinical trials of interferon-alfa and dacarbazine are underway for thick malignant melanomas.

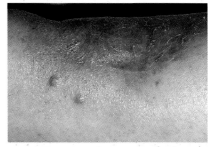

Fig. 10 **Hypomelanotic recurrent malignant melanoma.** The tumour has recurred at the edge of a previously excised and grafted site.

PREVENTION AND PUBLIC EDUCATION

Early malignant melanoma is a curable disease, but thick lesions have a poor prognosis. Public health education should encourage early visits to the doctor for changing pigmented lesions and should discourage excessive sun exposure, especially in fair-skinned individuals or those with numerous melanocytic naevi. The best advice is:

- avoid burning in the sun
- report early any change in a mole.

Malignant melanoma

- The UK incidence is 10 per 100 000 per year.
- The female to male ratio is 2:1.
- The incidence is rising by 7% per year and doubling every decade.
- The incidence is proportional to the geographic latitude, suggesting an effect of UV radiation.
- The prognosis is related to tumour thickness. Early lesions are curable by surgical excision.

MALIGNANT EPIDERMAL TUMOURS

Malignant skin tumours are amongst the most common of all cancers. They are more frequent in light-skinned races, and ultraviolet radiation seems to be involved in their aetiology. The incidence of *non-melanoma skin cancer* in caucasoids in the USA was recently estimated at 230 per 100000 per year, compared to 3 per 100000 for African-Americans. The majority of malignant skin tumours (Table 1) are epidermal in origin and are either basal cell or squamous cell carcinomas, or malignant melanomas (p. 94). Premalignant epidermal conditions are common (p. 98), but dermal malignancies are comparatively rare.

Table 1 **A classification of malignant skin tumours and premalignant conditions**

Cell origin	Premalignant condition	Malignant tumour
Keratinocyte	Actinic keratosis (p. 101) Intraepidermal carcinoma (p. 98)	Basal cell carcinoma Squamous cell carcinoma
Melanocyte	?Dysplastic naevus (p. 95)	Malignant melanoma (p. 94)
Fibroblast		Dermatofibrosarcoma (p. 98)
Lymphocyte		Lymphoma (p. 98)
Endothelium		Kaposi's sarcoma (p. 113)
Non-cutaneous		Secondary (p. 84)

BASAL CELL CARCINOMA

Basal cell carcinomas (rodent ulcers) are the commonest form of skin cancer and are seen typically on the face in elderly or middle-aged subjects. They arise from the basal keratinocytes of the epidermis, are locally invasive, but very rarely metastasize.

Aetiopathogenesis

Malignant transformation of basal cells may be induced by:

- prolonged ultraviolet exposure
- arsenic ingestion (e.g. in 'tonics')
- X-irradiation
- chronic scarring
- genetic predisposition (e.g. basal cell naevus syndrome).

Basal cell carcinomas are most common in caucasoids with a fair 'celtic' skin who live near the equator, and are seen more in males than in females. In the UK they mainly occur in those over the age of 40 years, although in Australia they may be seen in the 3rd decade.

Pathology

The tumour is classically composed of uniform basophilic cells, in well-defined islands, that invade the dermis from the epidermis as buds, lobules or strands (Fig. 1).

Clinical presentation

Basal cell carcinomas occur mainly on light-exposed sites, commonly around the nose, the inner canthus of the eyelids and the temple. They grow slowly but relentlessly, are locally invasive, and may destroy cartilage, bone and soft tissue structures. A lesion has often been present for 2 or more years before the patient seeks advice. Often more than one tumour is evident. There are four main types of basal cell carcinoma, all of which occasionally may be pigmented:

- *Nodular.* This is the commonest type of lesion and usually starts as

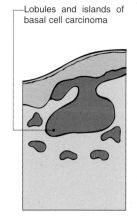

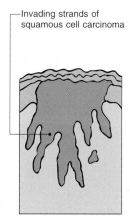

Fig. 1 **The histopathological structure of a basal cell carcinoma and a squamous cell carcinoma.**

Lobules and islands of basal cell carcinoma

Invading strands of squamous cell carcinoma

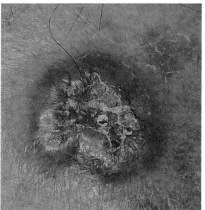

Fig. 2 **Basal cell carcinoma. The lesion shows the typical pearly edge, telangiectasia and central crusting.**

Fig. 3 **Basal call carcinoma of the nodular cystic type, occurring on the cheek adjacent to the nose.**

a small, skin-coloured papule which shows fine telangiectasia and a glistening pearly edge (Fig. 2). Central necrosis often occurs and leaves a small ulcer with an adherent crust. They are mostly less than 1cm in diameter, but grow larger if present for several years.

- *Cystic.* These become tense and translucent (Fig. 3), and show cystic spaces on histology.

- *Multicentric.* Superficial tumours, often multiple, plaque-like and several cm in diameter, are sometimes seen especially on the trunk. They have a rim-like edge and are frequently lightly pigmented.

- *Morphoeic.* This scarring (cicatricial) variant often shows a white or yellow morphoea-like plaque which may be centrally depressed.

Differential diagnosis

The differential diagnosis depends on the type and pigmentation of the basal cell carcinoma:

- *Nodular/cystic*: intradermal naevus (p. 92), molluscum contagiosum (p. 49), keratoacanthoma (p. 98), squamous cell carcinoma, sebaceous hyperplasia (a benign proliferation of sebaceous glands).
- *Multicentric*: discoid eczema (p. 34), psoriatic plaque (p. 26), intraepidermal carcinoma (p. 98).
- *Morphoeic*: morphoea (p. 77), scar.
- *Pigmented*: malignant melanoma (p. 94), seborrhoeic wart (p. 90), compound naevus (p. 92).

Management

The most appropriate treatment for any one tumour depends on its size, site, type and the patient's age. If possible, complete *excision* is the best treatment, since this allows a histological check on the adequacy of removal. If excision is difficult or not possible, incisional biopsy (to confirm the diagnosis) and *radiotherapy* are suitable for those aged 60 years and over. Large tumours around the eye and the nasolabial fold, especially if of the morphoeic type, are best managed by surgical excision. *Mohs microsurgery* (p. 105) may be employed, as these tumours are often more extensive than their appearance first suggests. *Curettage and cautery* is sometimes used for lesions on the trunk or upper extremities. *Cryosurgery* is an acceptable modality for multiple, superficial lesions, e.g. on the trunk.

The recurrence rate is about 5% at 5 years for most methods of treatment. Follow-up is particularly important if there is concern about the adequacy of removal.

SQUAMOUS CELL CARCINOMA

Squamous cell carcinoma is a malignant tumour, derived from keratinocytes, that usually arises in an area of damaged skin. It mainly occurs in people over 55 years of age, is more common in males than in females, and may metastasize.

Aetiopathogenesis

Squamous cell carcinoma is derived from moderately well-differentiated keratinocytes. Predisposing factors include:

- chronic actinic damage (p. 101)
- X-irradiation
- chronic ulceration and scarring
- smoking pipes and cigars (lip lesions)
- industrial carcinogens (tars, oils)
- wart virus and immunosuppression (p. 48)
- genetic (xeroderma pigmentosum, p. 89).

Pathology

The malignant keratinocytes, which retain the ability to produce keratin, destroy the dermo-epidermal junction and invade the dermis in an irregular manner (Fig. 1).

Clinical presentation

Squamous cell carcinomas usually develop in sun-exposed sites such as the face, neck, forearm or hand. The tumour may start within an actinic keratosis as a small papule which, if left, progresses to ulcerate and form a crust. This type of squamous cell carcinoma does not commonly metastasize. The nodular type of squamous cell carcinoma develops as a dome-shaped nodule sometimes, but not invariably, in sun-damaged skin (Fig. 4). Its shape differentiates it from

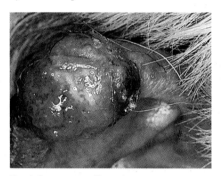

Fig. 4 **Squamous cell carcinoma.** The cancer is seen here on the upper pinna in a patient with actinically damaged skin.

the keratosis-derived variety. More aggressive ulcerating forms of squamous cell carcinoma are seen developing at the edge of ulcers (Fig. 5), in scars and at sites of radiation damage. Metastasis is found in 10% or more of these cancers.

Differential diagnosis

A squamous cell carcinoma needs to be distinguished from keratoacanthoma, actinic keratosis, basal cell carcinoma, intraepidermal carcinoma, amelanotic malignant melanoma and seborrhoeic keratosis. Excisional or incisional biopsy is needed in every case to confirm the diagnosis or adequacy of excision.

Management

Surgical excision is the treatment of choice. Large lesions may require a skin graft. In the elderly, squamous cell carcinomas of the face or scalp can be treated by *radiotherapy* (after an incisional biopsy for histological diagnosis). Patients are examined for lymph node metastasis at the time of presentation: suspicious nodes are biopsied.

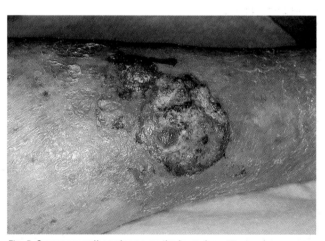

Fig. 5 **Squamous cell carcinoma on the lower leg.** The tumour occurred at the site of a long-standing ulcer.

Malignant epidermal tumours

- *Basal cell carcinoma* (rodent ulcer) is a common tumour often seen on the face in elderly or middle-aged patients. It:
  — is locally invasive
  — almost never metastasizes
  — is best treated by excision or sometimes incisional biopsy and radiotherapy.
- *Squamous cell carcinoma* in one form is found on sun-exposed sites in association with actinic keratoses and rarely metastasizes. Another type, seen with chronic scarring and ulceration, more commonly has metastases. All types are treated by excision.

PREMALIGNANT EPIDERMAL DISORDERS AND MALIGNANT DERMAL TUMOURS

Most premalignant epidermal conditions occur in sun-exposed sites, and ultraviolet radiation seems to play a role in their aetiology. Malignant tumours of the dermis are infrequent. The commonest causes are *secondary deposits* (p. 84), *Kaposi's sarcoma* (p. 52), a malignant tumour of dermal fibroblasts (*dermatofibrosarcoma*) and *cutaneous T-cell lymphoma*.

INTRAEPIDERMAL CARCINOMA (BOWEN'S DISEASE)

Intraepidermal carcinoma is common and typically occurs on the lower leg in elderly women. The lesions are solitary or multiple. Previous exposure to arsenicals predisposes to the condition.

Pink or lightly pigmented scaly plaques, up to several cm in size, are found on the lower leg or trunk (Fig. 1). Transformation into squamous cell carcinoma is infrequent. Intraepidermal carcinoma may resemble discoid eczema, psoriasis or superficial basal cell carcinoma. Histologically, the epidermis is thickened and the keratinocytes are atypical, but not invasive.

After histological confirmation, the abnormal area is treated by cryotherapy, curettage or excision.

KERATOACANTHOMA

A keratoacanthoma is a rapidly growing tumour usually arising in the sun-exposed skin of the face or arms (Fig. 2); it is not normally regarded as malignant. The tumour grows rapidly over a few weeks into a dome-shaped nodule up to 2 cm in diameter. There is often a keratin plug which may fall out to leave a crater. Spontaneous resolution will occur but takes several months and leaves an unpleasant scar.

Histologically, a keratoacanthoma may resemble a squamous cell carcinoma, although it shows more symmetry and shouldering. Excision is the preferred treatment, but thorough curettage and cautery will usually be satisfactory. If recurrence occurs after curettage, excision is recommended.

CUTANEOUS T-CELL LYMPHOMA (CTCL: MYCOSIS FUNGOIDES)

CTCL describes a lymphoma that evolves in the skin, although extra-

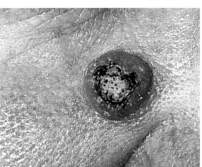

Fig. 2 **Keratoacanthoma on the face.**

cutaneous T-cell tumours often produce secondary skin deposits. CTCL is a slowly progressive tumour of CD 4+ lymphocytes which becomes systemic only in its terminal stage.

The course is usually protracted, although occasionally it is more rapidly progressive. The diagnosis may only be secured after repeated skin biopsy. CTCL can be regarded as having four stages, namely:

- *Premycotic plaques.* This phase is one type of parapsoriasis (p. 39) and resembles eczema or psoriasis. It may persist for 10 or more years. Occasionally the skin becomes atrophic, pigmented and telangiectatic (poikiloderma).
- *Infiltrated plaques.* Fixed plaques develop, usually on the trunk but sometimes more widely distributed (Fig. 3). This stage may last for years.
- *Tumour stage.* This late phase, characterized by tumorous nodules or ulcers within the plaques, has a mean survival of 2.5 years.
- *Systemic disease.* Involvement of lymph nodes or internal organs is a late finding. The Sézary syndrome (p. 40) is a variant of this phase.

Current treatment is not curative but aimed at controlling the lymphoma. The premycotic lesions often improve with moderately potent topical steroids and ultraviolet B therapy. More infiltrated plaques require PUVA, topical nitrogen mustard, photopheresis (p. 107) or electron-beam therapy. Localized nodules or tumours respond to conventional radiotherapy, but chemotherapy is disappointing.

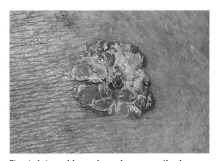

Fig. 1 **Intraepidermal carcinoma on the lower leg.**

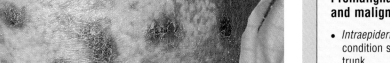

Fig. 3 **Cutaneous T-cell lymphoma showing infiltrated plaques and poikiloderma.**

Premalignant epidermal disorders and malignant dermal tumours

- *Intraepidermal carcinoma* is a common premalignant condition seen as a scaly plaque often on the lower leg or trunk.
- *Keratoacanthoma* is a rapidly growing dome-shaped tumour on the face or arm, which often shows a central keratin plug.
- *Cutaneous T-cell lymphoma* is an uncommon condition due to malignant T-lymphocytes. It progresses through stages of premycotic plaques and indurated plaques, finally to tumours and systemic involvement.

SPECIAL TOPICS
IN DERMATOLOGY

ULTRAVIOLET RADIATION AND THE SKIN

An interaction between skin and sunlight is inescapable. The potential for harm depends on the type and length of exposure. Photoageing is a growing problem, due to an increasingly aged population and a rise in the average individual exposure to UV radiation.

THE ELECTROMAGNETIC RADIATION SPECTRUM

The sun's emission of electromagnetic radiation ranges from low wavelength ionizing cosmic, gamma and X-rays to the non-ionizing ultraviolet (UV), visible and infrared higher wavelengths (Fig. 1). The ozone layer absorbs UVC, but UVA and smaller amounts of UVB reach ground level. UV radiation is maximum in the middle of the day (11 a.m. to 3 p.m.) and is increased by reflection from snow, water and sand. UVA penetrates the epidermis to reach the dermis. UVB is mostly absorbed by the stratum corneum — only 10% reaches the dermis. Most window glass absorbs UV less than 320 nm in wavelength. Artificial UV sources emit in the UVB or UVA spectrum. Sunbeds largely emit UVA.

EFFECTS OF LIGHT ON NORMAL SKIN

Physiological

UVB promotes the synthesis of vitamin D_3 from its precursors in the skin, and UVA and UVB stimulate immediate pigmentation (due to photo-oxidation of melanin precursors), melanogenesis and epidermal thickening as a protective measure against UV damage (p. 7).

Sunburn

If enough UVB is given, erythema always results. The threshold dose of UVB — the *minimal erythema dose* (MED) — is a guide to an individual's susceptibility. Excessive UVB exposure results in tingling of the skin followed 2–12 hours later by erythema. The redness is maximal at 24 hours and fades over the next 2 or 3 days to leave desquamation and pigmentation. Severe sunburn causes oedema, pain, blistering and systemic upset. The early use of topical steroids may help sunburn, otherwise a soothing shake lotion (e.g. calamine lotion) is applied. Individuals may be skin typed

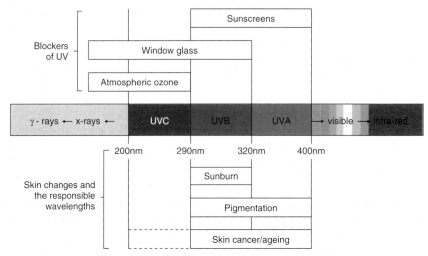

Fig. 1 **The sun's emission spectrum.**

Table 1 **Skin type according to sunburn/suntan**

Skin type	Reaction to sun exposure
Type 1	Always burns, never tans
Type 2	Always burns, sometimes tans
Type 3	Sometimes burns, always tans
Type 4	Never burns, always tans
Type 5	Brown skin (e.g. Asian caucasoid)
Type 6	Black skin (e.g. Black African)

by their likelihood of burning in the sun (Table 1). Prevention is better than cure, and Celts with a fair 'type 1' skin should not sunbathe and must use a high-protection-factor sunblock cream on exposed sites (p. 102).

Sunbeds

Sunbeds emit UVA radiation and have been used by 10–20% of adults in the UK. They will produce a tan in people with skin types 3 and over, but those with type 1 and 2 skin will not tan so well, if at all. Side-effects, particularly redness, itching and dry skin, are seen in a half of all users. More serious effects can occur in patients taking drugs or applying preparations with a photosensitizing potential. An acute photosensitive eruption may develop and intense pigmentation sometimes follows. Sunbeds can exacerbate polymorphic light eruption and systemic LE, and may induce porphyria-like skin fragility and blistering. They are a weak risk factor for malignant melanoma and animal studies suggest that they can cause premature skin ageing.

Dermatologists discourage use of sunbeds, particularly in the fair-skinned, those with several

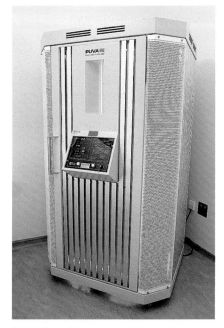

Fig. 2 **Photochemotherapy** using UVA-emitting tubes.

melanocytic naevi and in anyone with a history of skin cancer. Patients who, despite these warnings, wish to use a sunbed should not do so more than twice a year and should limit each course to 10 sessions. Sunbeds are not recommended for treatment of skin disease.

PHOTOTHERAPY AND PHOTOCHEMOTHERAPY

Natural sunlight helps certain skin diseases (p. 43) and both UVB and UVA are extensively used therapeutically. UVA alone has little effect and is combined with photosensitizing psoralens given systemically or topically.

Ultraviolet B

UVB (290–320 nm) is given 3 times a week. The starting dose is decided from the patient's MED or skin type. The dosage is increased each visit according to a schedule. A course of 10–30 treatments is usual. Narrow band (311–313 nm) UV lamps (p. 107) may have advantages but are still being evaluated.

UVB is used to treat psoriasis and mycosis fungoides and, occasionally, atopic eczema and pityriasis rosea. It can be given to children and women during pregnancy. Its main side effects are acute sunburn and an increased long-term risk of skin cancer.

When used to treat psoriasis, UVB may be combined with a topical preparation such as tar, dithranol or a vitamin D analogue (p. 28), or with oral acitretin.

Photochemotherapy (PUVA)

In *P*soralen plus *U*ltra*V*iolet *A* (PUVA) therapy, 8-methoxypsoralen, taken orally 2 hours before UVA (320–400nm) exposure (Fig. 2), is photoactivated, causing cross-linkage in DNA, inhibiting cell division and suppressing cell-mediated immunity. PUVA is usually given for psoriasis or mycosis fungoides, and sometimes for atopic eczema, polymorphic light eruption (p. 42) or vitiligo (p. 70). The initial dose of UVA is determined by the minimum toxic dose (the MED for PUVA) or skin type, and is increased according to a schedule. PUVA is given 2 or 3 times a week and leads to clearance of psoriasis (with tanning) in 15–25 treatments. Maintenance PUVA is not recommended. PUVA can be combined with acitretin ('RePUVA') but not methotrexate.

The immediate side-effects of pruritus, nausea and erythema are usually mild. The long-term risks of skin cancer and premature skin ageing are related to the number of treatments or total UVA dose. Careful records must be kept. Cataracts are theoretically possible, and UVA-opaque sunglasses must be worn for 24 hours after taking the psoralen.

Bath PUVA, in which the patient soaks in a bath containing a psoralen, is an alternative, especially if systemic side-effects make the oral route impractical. A lower dose of UVA is needed. *Local PUVA* using topical psoralen is useful for psoriasis or dermatitis of the hands or feet.

PHOTOAGEING

Photoageing describes the skin changes resulting from chronic sun exposure. Photoaged skin is coarse, wrinkled, pale-yellow in colour, telangiectatic, irregularly pigmented, prone to purpura and subject to benign and malignant neoplasms (Fig. 3). Some of these changes resemble those of intrinsic ageing, but the two are not identical as may be judged by comparing, in an elderly patient, the sun-exposed face with the sun-protected buttock. The features of photoageing are usually more striking, particularly the development of pre-malignant and malignant tumours. Some rare conditions, e.g. xeroderma pigmentosum (p. 89), predispose to photoageing.

Histologically, the photoaged dermis shows tangled clumps of elastin with proliferation of glycosaminoglycans (Fig. 4). The epidermis is variable in thickness, with areas of atrophy and hypertrophy and a variation in the degree of pigmentation. *In vitro*, keratinoctes and fibroblasts from sun-exposed sites have a reduced proliferative ability compared to cells from sun-protected sites.

Specific clinical changes of photoageing are discussed on page 111.

MANAGEMENT OF PHOTOAGEING

Prevention is the most effective treatment and is particularly important for those with a fair (type 1 or 2) skin. Avoidance of prolonged, direct sun exposure by wearing long-sleeved shirts and a wide-brimmed hat is useful, and sunscreens (p. 102) are applied to sites that are likely to receive some sun, such as the face or hands. The use of tretinoin or alpha hydroxy acids, in cream formulations, has been shown to partially reverse the clinical and histological changes of photoageing.

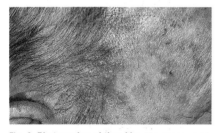

Fig. 3 **Photoageing of the skin.** Keratoses and pigmentation are evident.

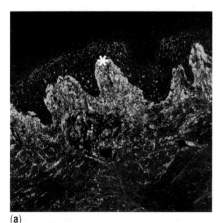

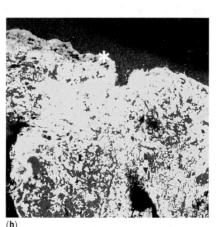

(a)   (b)

Fig. 4 (a) **Sun-protected skin** showing preservation of the normal pattern of glycosaminoglycan (GAG: green, hyaluronan) and fibriform elastin (red) (* shows dermoepidermal junction: DEJ).
(b) **Sun-exposed elastotic skin** showing tangled clumps of elastin (red), with proliferations of GAG (chondroitin sulphate) colocalized to elastin (yellow) throughout the dermis (* shows DEJ).

UV and the Skin

- *UVB radiation* is mostly absorbed by the epidermis, but UVA can penetrate to the dermis. UVB promotes vitamin D synthesis. UVA and UVB stimulate melanogenesis and epidermal thickening.
- *Minimal erythema dose* is the threshold of UVB to cause erythema.
- *Sunburn* is maximum at 24 hours and fades at 2–3 days to leave desquamation and pigmentation.
- *Sunbeds* emit UVA and will induce a tan in those with type 3 or 4 skin. Side-effects are common.
- *Photoageing* describes coarse, wrinkled, yellowed skin, prone to tumours, due to excess sun exposure.
- *UVB therapy* is mainly used in psoriasis: a course of 10–30 treatments is usual.
- *PUVA* is a popular treatment for psoriasis: skin cancer is a potential long-term sequela.
- *Treatment of photoageing:* prevention is best, but tretinoin cream can reverse some changes.

COSMETICS

A cosmetic may be defined as any substance that is applied to the body for cleansing, beautifying, promoting attractiveness or altering the appearance. Cosmetics in some form are used by almost everyone. The market for cosmetic sales is vast and far exceeding that of dermatological products. Over recent years the fields of cosmetology and dermatology have converged so that patients often present having had a reaction to a cosmetic or asking for advice about cosmetic usage. Some cosmetics are now being marketed with the claim that they have an 'active' ingredient, for example one which can 'reverse ageing'.

THE RANGE OF COSMETICS AND THEIR USAGE

Cosmetics are normally used to enhance the appearance of the body, to clean it, to impart a pleasing smell or mask an unpleasant one, or as a fashion accessory. Table 1 shows the range of common types of cosmetics.

Table 1 **The range of cosmetics**

Site	Product
Skin	Moisturiser, cleanser, soap, make-up remover, powder, rouge, foundation, 'tonic', perfume, aftershave, bath additive, sunscreen
Hair	Shampoo, conditioner, bleach, colourant, permanent waving, straightening, lacquer, gel, hair-removing agents
Eyelids	Mascara, eyeshadow, eyeliner, pencil
Nails	Nail varnish, varnish remover
Lips	Lipstick, lipgloss, sunscreen

CONSTITUENTS OF COSMETICS

The exact contents of a cosmetic depend on its proposed function. However, commonly used ingredients, some of which will be found in most cosmetics, are detailed in Table 2. Many cosmetics contain perfumes, preservatives, and, quite often, a sunblock agent. Cosmetics are often emulsions (e.g. oil-in-water or water-in-oil). Full labelling of contents is not yet required in the UK, although dermatologists are pressing for this to be introduced. Certain preparations deserve special mention and are discussed below.

Table 2 **Some ingredients of cosmetics**

Ingredient	Action	Examples
Oil, fat, wax	Emollient, lustre	Vaseline, almond oil, lanolin
Polyol	Humectant (retains water), emollient	Glycerol, propylene glycol, sorbitol
Tensio-active agent	Emulsifier, surfactant, detergent	Hydrophilic and hydrophobic molecules, soaps, stearic and oleic acids
Water	Hydration	Purified water
Preservative	Antimicrobial	Parabens, formaldehyde, Kathon CG, Dowicil 200, Bronopol, Germall 115
Anti-oxidant	Prevent degradation	Butylhydroxyanisole
Colourant, dye	Colour	Cochineal, azo compounds, iron dioxides, amino-phenol, PPD, titanium dioxide
Perfume	Smell or for masking smell	Balsam of Peru, eugenol
Sunfilter	Absorb or reflect UV	PABA, Eusolex 4360, Parsol 1789

Permanent waving agents

These are mostly reducing agents that break and reform the disulphide bonds between keratin chains in hair. Ammonium thioglycolate and glyceryl monothioglycolate are examples.

Nail preparations

Nail varnish is composed of a sulphonamide–formaldehyde resin and colourants. Artificial nails are made of methylmethacrylate and stuck on with acrylic glues.

Sunscreens

A sunscreen absorbs or reflects UV radiation. Absorbent agents are shown in Table 2. Titanium dioxide and zinc oxide are reflectant pigments. The protection factor indicates the ratio of the reaction time to erythema when exposed to UV radiation for treated as compared to untreated skin. Thus using a Factor 10 cream means that it should take 10 times longer for erythema to develop when in the sun. Some sunscreen creams are waterproof. Most need to be applied several times a day. Preparations available on prescription in the UK for patients with photodermatoses include RoC Total Sunblock, Spectraban 25, Sun E45, Uvistat Ultrablock and Piz Buin.

Camouflage cosmetics

These pigmented camouflage creams can be mixed to match the colour of the patient's skin and are useful for individuals who have vitiligo, disfiguring birthmarks or scars. Prescribable examples include Covermark and Dermacolor.

Skin lightening creams

These may contain mercury or hydroquinone, both of which can cause contact allergy or, paradoxically, pigmentation.

Hypoallergenic formulations

These cosmetics are made of highly purified ingredients, selected with the knowledge of their allergenic and irritant potential. However, they still contain compounds that are potential irritants and allergens.

REACTIONS TO COSMETICS

Side-effects are comparatively rare when the vast usage of cosmetics is considered but, none the less, 12% or more of adults have had a reaction to a cosmetic. Some responses, e.g. stinging with aftershave due to the alcohol base, are expected and do not constitute a reaction. The preparations most likely to cause a problem are eye and facial cosmetics, antiperspirants and deodorants, hair colourants and soaps (Table 3). Reactions can be categorized as follows.

Table 3 **Frequent adverse reactions to cosmetics**

Cosmetic	Reaction
Soap, detergent	Mostly irritant
Deodorant, antiperspirant	Irritant, sometimes allergic
Moisturiser	Irritant and allergic
Eyeshadow	Mostly irritant
Mascara	Mostly irritant
Permanent wave	Irritant and allergic
Hair dye	Allergic
Shampoo	Mostly irritant

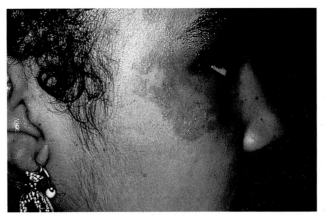

Fig. 1 **Irritant contact dermatitis to a component of a hair-removing cream.**

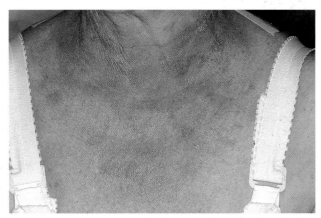

Fig. 2 **Allergic contact dermatitis on the neck due to fragrances.**

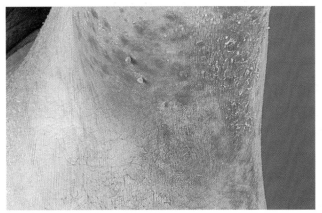

Fig. 3 **Allergic contact dermatitis at the axilla to a component of a cream.**

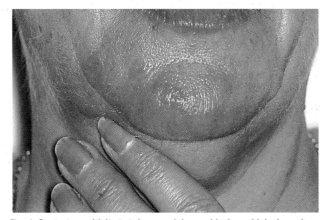

Fig. 4 **Contact sensitivity to toluene sulphonamide-formaldehyde resin in nail varnish, causing a facial dermatitis.**

Irritant contact dermatitis

This is particularly seen in atopics and those with a 'sensitive' skin. Soaps, which are drying and alkaline (the normal pH of facial skin is about 5.5), and deodorants cause mostly irritant dermatitis (Fig. 1). Lanolins, detergents and preservatives may also be irritant.

Allergic contact sensitivity

Allergic contact dermatitis most commonly develops to fragrances, preservatives, dyes (e.g. paraphenylenediamine — PPD), lanolins and glyceryl monothioglycolate (Figs 2 & 3). The eruption usually develops at the place of application of the product (usually the face), but this is not always so, as substances can be transferred to another site where they cause symptoms. For example, contact allergy to sulphonamide–formaldehyde resin (Fig. 4) in nail varnish most often manifests as an eruption around the eyelids or on the neck.

Contact urticaria and other adverse reactions

Contact urticaria presents as a wheal and flare response within a few minutes of the application of a substance. It may occur with compounds in perfumes, shampoos and hair dyes.

Other adverse reactions include nail dystrophies caused by nail cosmetic use, hair breakage and weathering due to improper use of permanent waving, hair straighteners or dyes, pigmentation and acne.

MANAGEMENT OF COSMETIC REACTIONS

A patient intolerant of a cosmetic should stop the use of all cosmetics and, if necessary, be treated with a topical steroid until the reaction subsides. All the cosmetics and preparations that have been used must be examined, and patch testing (p. 118) performed if appropriate. Alternative cosmetics can then be introduced, but kept to a minimum.

Cosmetics

- A *cosmetic* is a substance applied to the body for cleansing, to promote attractiveness or to alter the appearance.
- A *cosmetic cream* typically contains emollients, emulsifiers, colourants, perfumes, and preservatives to prevent oxidation and the growth of microorganisms. Sunfilters may also be included.
- *Reactions to cosmetics* may take the form of irritant or allergic contact dermatitis, or contact urticaria.
- The commonest causes of *irritant reactions* are soaps, shampoos and deodorants, often due to detergents or preservatives.
- The substances that most frequently cause *allergic contact dermatitis* are fragrances, or preservatives (found in most cosmetics, e.g. moisturisers), and dyes (e.g. as found in hair colourants).

BASIC DERMATOLOGICAL SURGERY

The demand for the removal of benign and malignant skin lesions has increased considerably such that skin surgery is now practised by many general practitioners as well as by dermatologists. A knowledge of basic surgical techniques is mandatory for all those who treat skin disease.

INSTRUMENTS AND METHODS

No-one should attempt a procedure if unsure about it. Those with limited experience should remove only benign lesions. All procedures are ideally performed in an *operating theatre* with trained nurses and adequate lighting. Sterile instruments, an aseptic technique and sterile gloves are essential. The operator plans the procedure, explains it to the patient, obtains written consent and discusses the scar. The direction of crease marks is assessed: any excision is usually made parallel to these lines.

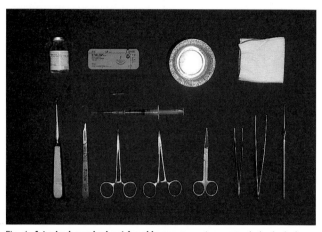

Fig. 1 **A typical surgical set for skin surgery.** A curette is included.

The *basic instruments* (Fig. 1) include a #3 scalpel handle and #15 blade, a toothed Adsons forceps, a small smooth-jawed needle-holder, a pair of fine scissors, artery forceps and a Gillies skin hook. Curettes and skin punches come in various sizes. A solution of 1% lignocaine (Xylocaine) with 1 in 200 000 adrenaline is usually satisfactory as the *local anaesthetic*, but plain lignocaine must be used on the fingers, toes and penis. The skin is prepared (but not sterilized) using, e.g. 0.075% aqueous chlorhexidine (Savlodil). Alcohol-based preparations are avoided as, if cautery is used, the solution may ignite. Sterile towels, placed around the operation site, reduce the chance of infection.

The commonest *suture materials* are silk and nylon. Silk is the easiest to handle and best for beginners, but nylon, although more difficult to tie, gives less of a tissue reaction and leaves fewer marks. Use 5/0 sutures

on the face, 3/0 on the back and legs, and 4/0 elsewhere. Stitches are preferably removed at 5 days on the face, 10–14 days on the legs or back, and 7–8 days at other sites. Steristrips give extra support to a wound either in addition to sutures, or when applied after their removal. A non-adherent dressing is used if necessary.

Every lesion biopsied is sent for histology. If more than one specimen is taken from a patient, separate pots are used and each labelled before the biopsy is placed in it. The usual fixative is 10% formalin.

BASIC SURGICAL TECHNIQUES

Excisional biopsy

An excisional biopsy is planned after considering the local anatomy. The excision's axis depends on the skin creases (Fig. 2) and its margin on the nature of the lesion. The ellipse to be excised is drawn on the skin using a

marker pen. An ellipse has an apical angle of about 30 degrees and is usually three times as long as it is wide. If any shorter, 'dog-ears' appear at either end, though these can easily be removed. After cleaning, local anaesthetic is infiltrated, using a fine needle, into the area of the lesion. Once numbed, the skin is incised vertically down to fat with the scalpel, in a smooth continuous manner to complete both arcs of the ellipse. The ellipse is freed from surrounding skin, secured at one end with a skin hook and removed from the underlying fat, usually using the scalpel blade (Fig. 3). In most cases the wound can now be repaired, although first any bleeding vessels will need to be tied off.

In a simple *interrupted skin suture*, the needle is inserted vertically through the skin surface down through the dermis and up the other side of the incision to trace a flask-shaped profile (Fig. 3). The wound is

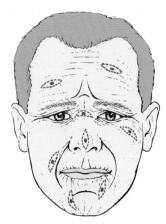

Fig. 2 **Facial crease lines, with some examples of excision ellipses.**

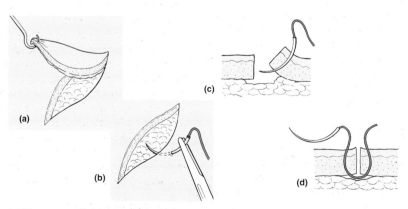

Fig. 3 **Ellipse removal and suture insertion. (a)** The ellipse is removed, one end being secured with a skin hook. **(b)** The suture needle is inserted vertically through the skin surface. **(c)** The suture needle pierces the full thickness of the epidermis and dermis. **(d)** The tied suture is 'flask' shaped and slightly everts the skin surface.

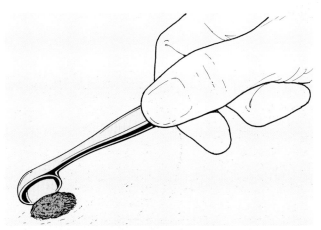

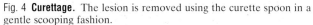

Fig. 4 **Curettage.** The lesion is removed using the curette spoon in a gentle scooping fashion.

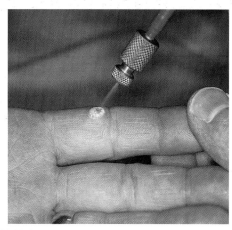

Fig. 5 **Liquid nitrogen treatment using a cryotherapy apparatus.**

apposed and slightly everted. Stitches should not be tied too tightly. Silk is knotted twice on the first throw and once on the two subsequent throws. Nylon usually needs three knots on the first and two on the two subsequent throws. Throws in alternating directions produce a square knot. Care is exercised at sites where keloids may form (e.g. the upper back, chest or jawline), where scars may be obvious (e.g. the face of a young woman) and when healing may be poor (e.g. the lower leg). Absorbable subcutaneous sutures are used for big excisions.

Incisional, punch and shave biopsies

An *incisional biopsy* is done for diagnostic purposes. The technique is similar to an excision except that less tissue is taken. A *punch biopsy* employs a punch (normally about 4 mm in diameter), which is twisted into the skin: the resultant cylinder of skin is removed and the defect cauterized or repaired with a single suture. *Shave biopsy* is employed for benign lesions, usually intradermal naevi or seborrhoeic warts. The lesion is shaved off parallel to, but slightly above, the skin surface. Haemostasis is achieved with cautery. Not all the lesion is removed and shaving is not used if malignancy is a possibility. Skin tags are removed by simply snipping them off with scissors and cauterizing any bleeding points.

Curettage

Curettage is performed for seborrhoeic warts, pyogenic granulomas, keratoacanthomas or single viral warts (e.g. on the face) but not for naevi. After being anaesthetized, the lesion is removed by a gentle scooping motion with the curette spoon (Fig. 4), and then the base is cauterized.

OTHER SURGICAL TECHNIQUES

Cautery

Cautery secures haemostasis and destroys tissue. The conventional cautery machine has an electrically-heated wire and is self-sterilizing. The *Birtcher Hyfrecator*, a unipolar diathermy, gives better controlled electrocautery. It can be used to treat spider naevi and telangiectasia, and to give haemostasis, but is contraindicated in patients with cardiac pacemakers. Silver nitrate sticks or 35% aluminium chloride in 50% isopropyl alcohol provide chemical cautery.

Cryotherapy

Cryotherapy using liquid nitrogen is effective for viral warts, molluscum contagiosum, seborrhoeic warts, actinic keratoses, intraepidermal carcinoma and, in some instances, biopsy-proven basal cell carcinoma. The liquid nitrogen (at $-196°C$) is delivered by cotton wool bud or spray gun (e.g. Cry-Ac) and injures cells by ice formation. After immersion in a flask containing liquid nitrogen, a cotton wool bud on a stick is applied to the lesion for about 10 seconds until a thin frozen halo appears at the base. The spray gun is used from a distance of about 10 mm for a similar length of freeze (Fig. 5). Longer freeze-times are given for malignant tumours. Blisters may develop within 24 hours. They are punctured and a dry dressing applied. Side-effects include hypopigmentation of pigmented skin and ulceration of lower leg lesions, particularly in the elderly. Treatment is repeated after 4 weeks if necessary.

Specialized procedures

Mohs' surgery describes the serial excision of a malignant tumour, which is mapped and examined microscopi-

cally to define its extent and the adequacy of excision. A *flap* is a specialized method of wound closure by moving the surrounding skin. *Dermabrasion*, sometimes suggested for scars, involves a rotating mechanical head which wounds the skin down to the dermis. *Lasers* (*Light Amplification by Stimulated Emission of Radiation*) apply a very high intensity light energy to the tissue and are useful for port wine stain naevi, telangiectasia, tattoos, viral warts and some tumours (p. 107).

Dermatological surgery

- *Skin surgery* is best performed in an operating theatre with aseptic technique, adequate lighting and trained nurses.
- 1% lignocaine with 1/200 000 adrenaline is an adequate *local anaesthetic* for most sites.
- *Silk sutures* are easy to handle, but *nylon* gives fewer stitch marks.
- All biopsy material is sent for *histology*.
- *Excisions* are done as an ellipse, parallel to the crease marks, and are about three times as long as wide.
- *Shave biopsy* is suitable for removal of benign naevi.
- *Curettage* is a good treatment for seborrhoeic warts, single viral warts, and pyogenic granulomas.
- *Cautery* secures haemostasis and destroys tissue.
- *Cryotherapy* is used for viral and seborrhoeic warts, premalignant conditions and some tumours.
- *Lasers* are useful for port wine stain naevi.

NEW TRENDS IN DERMATOLOGICAL TREATMENT

Therapeutic advances have revolutionized the treatment of skin disease over the last 30 years. The 1960s saw the introduction of topical steroids, the 1970s witnessed the development of PUVA and in the 1980s, the retinoids were introduced to clinical practice. The most recent improvements, outlined below, although not of comparable significance, represent advances for certain conditions.

There have also been improvements in the delivery of care. Over the last few years the number of in-patient dermatology beds has dropped dramatically, and patients who would have been admitted are now managed in *day-care units*. Dermatological nursing skills have been transferred to the out-patient setting, resulting in a higher profile for nurse practitioners who often run their own clinics, e.g. for patients with leg ulcers, eczema or psoriasis.

ACNE

The topical application of *nicotinamide* (Papulex), *azelaic acid* (Skinoren) and *isotretinoin* (Isotrex) are effective for mild-to-moderate acne. *Combination* topical treatments, such as erythromycin and zinc acetate (Zineryt) or erythromycin and benzoyl peroxide (Benzamycin), may offer some advantage for mild-to-moderate acne.

ATOPIC ECZEMA

Patients with atopic eczema, particularly children and their parents, benefit from counselling by a specialist nurse. A full explanation of the condition, day-to-day aspects of management and advice on topical therapy are very helpful and provide much needed support and reassurance.

Staphylococcus aureus nearly always colonizes the skin in atopic eczema and may, through its action as a *super-antigen*, non-specifically activate T-cells which release cytokines and cause inflammation. This is the rationale for treatments aimed at reducing skin carriage of staphylococci, e.g. *mupirocin* (Bactroban) or *fusidic acid* (Fucidin) ointments or creams, and antiseptic bath additives such as Emulsiderm or Oilatum Plus.

Second-line treatments for atopic eczema include ultraviolet B (UVB), PUVA, cyclosporin, azathioprine and *Chinese herbal remedies*. The traditional Chinese treatment consists of about 10 herbs given in the form of a 'tea'. It is effective in some patients but may cause liver problems, and is rather inconvenient to take as it must be brewed up each day.

The mainstay of topical treatment in atopic eczema remains *emollients* and *steroids*. Recently introduced 'new' generation topical corticosteroids, such as *fluticasone* (Cutivate) or *mometasone* (Elocon), have a better safety profile than previous steroids, i.e. they cause less skin atrophy (Fig. 1) and adrenal suppression, and have the added advantage of once-daily application.

FUNGAL INFECTIONS

Pulse treatment with *itraconazole* (Sporanox) has given cure rates of 80% for fungal infection (Fig. 2) of the toenails. The pulse consists of itraconazole 200mg twice daily for 7 days followed by a 3 week drug-free interval. This course is taken twice for fingernail infections and three times for infected toenails.

Terbinafine (Lamisil) cream, applied once or twice daily for one week, can cure tinea pedis (Fig. 3). Tinea capitis (Fig. 4) always requires systemic therapy.

HERPES ZOSTER AND HERPES SIMPLEX

Famciclovir, 250mg 3 times daily for 7 days, is effective in herpes zoster and may reduce post-herpetic neuralgia. It can also be used in genital herpes simplex. Topical *capsaicin* (Axsain) relieves post-herpetic neuralgia by depleting dermal nerves of substance P.

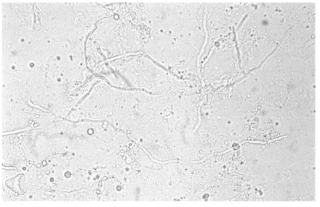

Fig. 2 **Fungal hyphae shown on microscopy.**

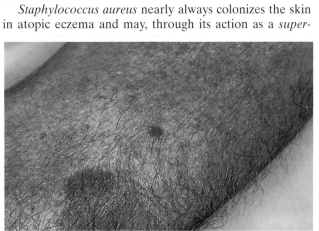

Fig. 1 **Skin atrophy with purpura due to excessive topical use of a potent steroid.**

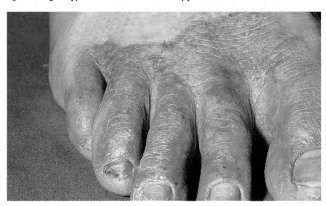

Fig. 3 **Tinea pedis.**

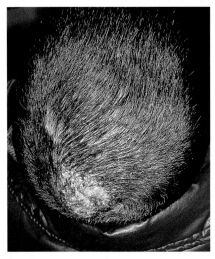

Fig. 4 Kerion with associated alopecia. The boggy pustular lesion results from a zoophilic fungal infection (p. 63).

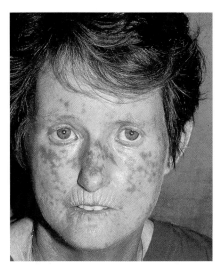

Fig. 5 Systemic sclerosis of the face. Telangiectasia and furrowing around the mouth are prominent changes.

LASERS

The technology of *lasers* (*L*ight *A*mplification by *S*timulated *E*mission of *R*adiation) has advanced rapidly, and lasers can now be used to treat vascular or pigmented lesions, various tumours, and tattoos. The variation in

Table 1 **The application of commonly-used lasers**

Laser	Wavelength	Application
Flashlamp short-pulsed dye	510 nm	Pigmented lesions e.g. lentigines, freckles, red tattoos
Nd-YAG Q-switched	532 nm	Pigmented lesions; adult port-wine stains, black/blue tattoos
Flashlamp long-pulsed dye	585 nm	Port-wine stains in children, warts, telangiectasia, hypertrophic scars
Alexandrite Q-switched	755 nm	Multicoloured tattoos, naevus of Ota, viral warts
Carbon dioxide continuous/pulsed	10 600 nm	Tissue destruction, epidermal naevi, warts, tumours, rhinophyma

absorption of different wavelengths of light means that more than one type of laser is needed to treat different lesions. (Table 1). Treatment should be carried out in specialized centres. Several visits are usually required.

LEG ULCERS

Allergic contact dermatitis is common in patients with leg ulcers and preservatives in bandages are often responsible. A preservative-free *zinc paste bandage* (Steripaste) is now available. In patients with non-healing leg ulcers, *skin equivalents* consisting of cultured keratinocytes on dermis may be grafted onto the wound.

Venous leg ulcers are treated primarily by compression, preferably using the four-layer technique. A new type of *compression bandage* (Surepress) may allow adequate compression with less than four layers.

PSORIASIS

Narrow band (311–313 nm) UVB may have some advantages over broadband UVB or PUVA in the treatment of patients with psoriasis. *Calcipotriol* (Dovonex) is a well established first-line topical treatment for psoriasis, and now a further vitamin D analogue, *tacalcitol* (Curatoderm), has been introduced. Tacalcitol can be applied to the face and is effective once daily.

New, receptor-selective, topical

retinoids may soon be available for psoriasis. One example, *tazarotene*, binds skin retinoic acid receptors, modulating keratinocyte proliferation and inflammatory markers.

SKIN CANCER

Photodynamic therapy involves the topical application of the porphyrin precursor 5-amino-laevulinic acid to a lesion which is then irradiated with visible or laser light. It is very effective in intraepidermal carcinoma, actinic keratoses and superficial basal cell carcinoma. Intralesional injections of *interferon-gamma* may be used to treat certain basal cell carcinomas.

SYSTEMIC SCLEROSIS

Dihydroxycholecalciferol inhibits collagen synthesis and has been shown to be of benefit in systemic sclerosis (Fig. 5). *Photophoresis* (see below) and *PUVA* may also be helpful.

T-CELL LYMPHOMA

Currently, the combination of *acitretin* (Neotigason) and *interferon-alfa* is under evaluation. *Photophoresis*, in which a lymphocyte-enriched blood fraction from the patient, who has taken a psoralen, is exposed to UVA outside the body and then re-infused, is sometimes effective, especially for the Sézary syndrome (p. 98).

New trends in dermatological treatment

Disease	Topical therapy	Systemic therapy
Acne	Combination topicals, azelaic acid, nicotinamide	
Atopic eczema	Mupirocin, fusidic acid, fluticasone, mometasone	Cyclosporin, PUVA
Fungal	Terbinafine	Pulse itraconazole (for onychomycosis)
Herpes zoster	Famciclovir	Capsaicin (for neuralgia)
Leg ulcers	Surepress bandage (compression), Steripaste zinc bandage	
Psoriasis	Vitamin D analogues (calcipotriol/tacalcitol)	Narrow-band UVB
Skin cancer	Photodynamic therapy	Intralesional interferon-gamma (for basal cell carcinoma)
Systemic sclerosis		Dihydroxycholecalciferol, photophoresis, PUVA
T-cell lymphoma		Acitretin/interferon-alfa, photophoresis

PAEDIATRIC DERMATOLOGY

Some conditions are almost exclusive to childhood (e.g. napkin dermatitis and juvenile plantar dermatosis) and others are more common in children (e.g. atopic eczema or viral exanthems). The common childhood dermatoses not mentioned elsewhere are detailed here along with some rare but important disorders.

CHILDHOOD ECZEMAS AND RELATED DISORDERS

Forms of eczema found in childhood include:

- napkin dermatitis
- infantile seborrhoeic dermatitis
- candidiasis
- juvenile plantar dermatosis
- napkin psoriasis (p. 27)
- atopic eczema (p. 32)
- pityriasis alba (p. 39).

NAPKIN (DIAPER) DERMATITIS

Napkin dermatitis is the commonest type of napkin eruption. It is usually seen in infants who are only a few weeks old, and is rare after the age of 12 months. It is an irritant dermatitis due to the macerating effect of prolonged contact of the skin with faeces and urine, and the moisture retention caused by the use of plastic pants. A glazed erythema is seen in the napkin area, sparing the skin folds. Erosions or ulceration may follow (Fig. 1), and hypopigmentation is a complication in pigmented skin. Secondary bacterial or *C. albicans* infection is frequent, and the latter may account for the development of erythematous papules or pustules.

The *differential diagnosis* is from infantile seborrhoeic eczema and candidiasis, both of which tend to affect the flexures. The treatment of napkin dermatitis is aimed at keeping the area dry. The use of disposable super-absorbent nappies helps. A bland preparation such as aqueous cream is used as an emollient and soap substitute, and a silicone-based cream (e.g. Drapolene) may have a protective action. Topical 1% hydrocortisone, with an antifungal (e.g. Daktacort or Canesten-HC creams), is also effective.

INFANTILE SEBORRHOEIC ECZEMA

Infantile seborrhoeic eczema starts in the first few weeks of life and tends to affect the body folds, including the axillae, groin and neck, but it also may involve the face and scalp. Flexural lesions present as moist, shiny well-demarcated scaly erythema (Fig. 2), but on the scalp a yellowish crust is often found. The condition can usually be differentiated from *napkin dermatitis* (which spares the flexures), *candidiasis* (which is usually pustular) and *atopic eczema* (which is more pruritic). Infantile seborrhoeic eczema is treated by emollients and 1% hydrocortisone ointment, or with a hydrocortisone antifungal combination. Scalp lesions respond to 2% salicylic acid in aqueous cream applied once daily and washed out with a baby shampoo. Olive oil or arachis oil will help soften the scalp scales of cradle cap.

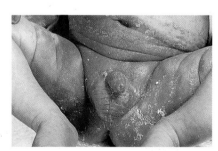
Fig. 2 **Infantile seborrhoeic eczema.** The condition involves the flexures.

CANDIDIASIS

Primary infection with *C. albicans* is unusual in a healthy infant; it is more common for the organism to secondarily complicate infantile seborrhoeic eczema or napkin dermatitis. Erythema, scaling and pustules are seen, often involving the flexures, and there may be satellite lesions. Treatment is with a topical antifungal agent such as Canesten, Daktarin, Ecostatin or Exelderm.

JUVENILE PLANTAR DERMATOSIS

Juvenile plantar dermatosis, first recognized in the 1970s, presents with red, dry, fissured and glazed skin, principally over the forefeet but sometimes involving the whole sole (Fig. 3). It usually starts in the primary school years and resolves spontaneously in the early to mid-teens. The condition is thought to be linked to the wearing of socks and shoes made from synthetic materials, although it may be a manifestation of atopy in some children. It is usual to advise cotton socks and less occlusive footwear — preferably made of leather. Topical steroids are ineffective but emollients help.

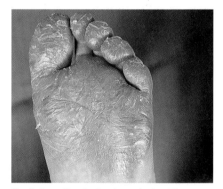
Fig. 3 **Juvenile plantar dermatosis.** The forefoot is mainly affected.

OTHER CHILDHOOD DERMATOSES

Some uncommon but characteristic eruptions are found in childhood. These include:

- urticaria pigmentosa
- histiocytosis-X
- Kawasaki disease and other viral infections (p. 49)
- ichthyosis (p. 86)
- epidermolysis bullosa (p. 87).

URTICARIA PIGMENTOSA

Urticaria pigmentosa is characterized by multiple reddish-brown macules or papules on the trunk and limbs of an infant. The lesions may become red, swollen, and itchy after a bath or when

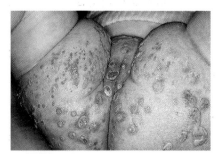
Fig. 1 **Napkin dermatitis.** A severe erosive variant is seen here.

rubbed, and blistering may occur. Histologically, there are accumulations of mast cells in the dermis. The disorder normally resolves spontaneously before adolescence. There is a form with a later onset, usually beginning in adolescence or adult life. It rarely resolves and may involve internal organs — something rare in the childhood variety.

HISTIOCYTOSIS-X (LANGERHANS CELL HISTIOCYTOSIS)

Histiocytosis-X is a rare and serious condition which normally involves internal organs. The skin signs are common, variable and include a seborrhoeic-like dermatitis, papules or pustules on the trunk and ulceration, particularly of the flexures. The skin, abdominal organs, lungs and bones are infiltrated by Langerhans cells which may behave in a malignant fashion, although the condition is believed to be a hyperplasia and not a true malignancy. Skin biopsy is usually diagnostic. The prognosis is poor when the onset is before 2 years of age.

VASCULAR NAEVI

Vascular naevi are common and are present at birth or develop soon after. Superficial lesions are due to capillary networks in the upper or mid dermis, but larger angiomas show multiple vascular channels in the lower dermis and subcutis.

CLINICAL PRESENTATION

There are four main clinical pictures which are described below.

Salmon patch

This is the commonest vascular naevus, seen in about 50% of neonates. Patches at the upper eyelid fade quickly, but the 'stork-mark' at the posterior neck often persists.

Port-wine stain naevus

Present at birth, the port-wine stain (or *naevus flammeus*) is an irregular red or purple macule which often affects one side of the face (Fig. 4). In middle age it can darken and become lumpy. A port-wine stain involving the trigeminal nerve's ophthalmic division may have an associated intracranial vascular malformation (the *Sturge–Weber syndrome*).

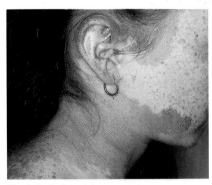

Fig. 4 **Port-wine stain naevus.**

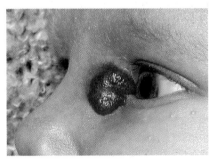

Fig. 5 **Strawberry naevus in an infant.**

Strawberry naevus

Also known as a capillary-cavernous haemangioma, this lesion usually develops during the first few weeks of life and grows to reach its maximum in the first 12 months (Fig. 5). It remains static for the next 6–12 months and then involutes; most cases will have regressed by the age of 5–7 years, leaving an area of atrophy. They occur anywhere on the skin surface.

Cavernous haemangioma

Similar to a strawberry naevus, this is composed of larger and deeper vascular channels and presents as a nodular swelling. The overlying skin may be normal or show a superficial vascular component. Regression is not as complete as in a strawberry naevus. Large haemangiomas may trap platelets and cause thrombocytopenia (the *Kasabach–Merritt syndrome*).

MANAGEMENT

Port-wine stains may be covered with camouflage cosmetics (p. 102), but treatment is now available with the pulsed tunable dye laser (p. 107), which obliterates the abnormal dermal vessels and improves the appearance. Strawberry naevi should be allowed to involute unless they compromise vital structures such as the eye or airway. In this case a short course of prednisolone or even emergency surgery is needed. The Kasabach–Merritt syndrome is treated in a similar fashion.

Paediatric dermatology

Disorder	Age at onset	Clinical features
Napkin dermatitis	First few weeks to 12 months	Glazed erythema that spares body folds. Erosions may occur
Infantile seborrhoeic eczema	First few weeks	Moist scaly erythema. Flexures and scalp affected
Candidiasis	Infancy	Erythema, with scaling and pustules. Flexures affected. Secondary infection found
Juvenile plantar dermatosis	School age to mid-teens	Glazed red fissured skin on the forefeet and soles
Urticaria pigmentosa	Mostly at 3–9 months	Reddish-brown macules or papules on trunk, which urticate when rubbed
Histiocytosis-X	All ages (different types)	Seborrhoeic-like dermatitis, papules/pustules, ulceration
Vascular naevi	At birth, in first few weeks	Salmon patch on neck, port-wine naevus (e.g. on face), strawberry naevus

THE SKIN IN OLD AGE

In Western countries the proportion of people aged over 65 is high and continues to rise. Poor nutrition, lack of self care and general illness contribute to skin disease in the elderly. Few people die from old skin but many suffer from it.

INTRINSIC AGEING OF THE SKIN

The changes in aged, sun-protected skin are more subtle than those of photoageing (p. 101) and consist of laxity, fine wrinkling and benign neoplasms. In addition, androgenetic alopecia (p. 62) and greying of the hair are age related.

Histologically, the epidermis is thinned with the loss of the rete ridge pattern and a reduction in the numbers of melanocytes and Langerhans cells. Individual epidermal cells are smaller. The dermis is thinned due, mainly, to loss of proteoglycans. Functionally, the skin is less elastic and has a reduced tensile strength. Resistance to injury, irritants and infection is reduced and wound healing is slower.

Some inherited disorders, e.g. pseudoxanthoma elasticum (p. 89), show features of aged skin. The misuse of potent topical steroids induces atrophy and purpura (p. 66), signs also seen in old skin.

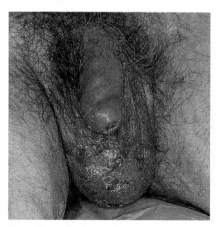

Fig. 1 **Flexural seborrhoeic** dermatitis affecting the scrotum and penis.

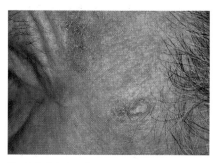

Fig. 3 **Actinic keratoses.**

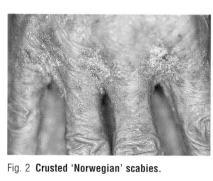

Fig. 2 **Crusted 'Norwegian' scabies.**

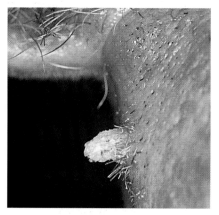

Fig. 4 **A cutaneous horn.**

DERMATOSES IN THE ELDERLY

Few skin conditions are exclusive to old age but some are seen more frequently (Table 1).

DRY SKIN AND ASTEATOTIC ECZEMA

Dryness with itching is common in elderly skin. It may be a mild roughness and scaling, or more severe, with fissuring and inflammation (asteatotic eczema p. 35). The changes often occur on the legs and are aggravated by low humidity, central heating and excessive washing. Emollients, sometimes with a mild or moderate-potency topical steroid ointment, usually help.

Seborrhoeic dermatitis (p. 34) in the elderly (Fig. 1) may be flexural and resemble psoriasis, candidiasis or erythrasma. In old people, *allergic contact dermatitis* (p. 30) tends to occur to allergens in topical medicaments or bandages, e.g. lanolins, neomycin, local anaesthetics and rubber chemicals.

Table 1 **Skin disorders common in the elderly**

The eczemas	Asteatotic/dry skin (p. 35) Seborrhoeic (p. 34) Contact (p. 32) Venous (p. 34)	Benign tumours	Seborrhoeic wart (p. 90) Cherry angioma (p. 91) Skin tag (p. 90) Chondrodermatitis nodularis
Other eruptions	Psoriasis (p. 26) Drug eruption (p. 82) Erythema ab igne (p. 67)	Photodamage	Photoageing (p. 101) Actinic elastosis
Infections	Herpes zoster (p. 51) Candidiasis (p. 55) Onychomycosis (p. 64) Scabies (p. 59)	Premalignant	Actinic keratosis Intraepidermal carcinoma (p. 98)
		Cancers	Basal cell carcinoma (p. 96) Squamous cell carcinoma (p. 97) Lentigo malignant melanoma (p. 94) Cutaneous T cell lymphoma (p. 98)
Ulceration	Leg ulcer (p. 68) Pressure ulcer	Other	Senile pruritus
Autoimmune	Pemphigoid (p. 74)		

PRURITUS

Itch in old age can be severe and unrelenting. Examination will usually show asteatotic eczema, scabies, urticaria or the pre-bullous phase of pemphigoid (p. 74), or investigations may reveal renal or liver disease or underlying malignancy (p. 85). The small group of patients in whom no cause is found have 'senile pruritus'. Topical treatments and sedating antihistamines often are ineffective.

PSORIASIS

Psoriasis has its peak onset in the teens with a second peak in the sixth decade. In the elderly patient, it is frequently flexural (p. 27) but all patterns, except guttate, are seen. Management can be difficult due to inability to apply topical therapy, attend hospital, or stand for UV treatment. Methotrexate is quite often used and is mostly well tolerated.

INFECTIONS AND INFESTATIONS

Herpes zoster (p. 51) at some time affects 25% of people over 65. Post-herpetic neuralgia increases with age, occurring in 75% of shingles victims over 70. Early treatment with aci-clovir, famciclovir (p. 106) or prednisolone makes neuralgia less likely.

Infection with *Candida albicans* (p. 55) is common in the flexures of obese elderly women. *Onychomycosis* (p. 64) is a frequent incidental finding in old people, especially men. Treatment is not always needed unless the nail produces pain.

Scabies epidemics are a problem in old people's homes and are difficult to control (p. 59). Any itchy old person

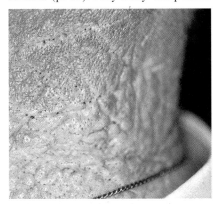

Fig. 5 **Actinic elastosis.** The characteristic rhomboid pattern is seen on the neck, associated with senile comedones.

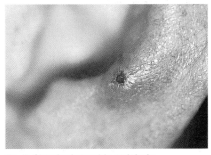

Fig. 6 **Chondrodermatitis nodularis.**

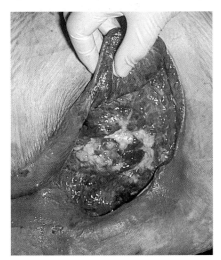

Fig. 7 **Pressure ulcer over the sacrum.**

should be examined carefully, as burrows are easily missed. Elderly patients who are debilitated, paralysed, immunosuppressed or who cannot scratch may develop crusted 'Norwegian' scabies (Fig. 2) which is highly contagious due to the thousands of mites present.

PHOTODAMAGE AND SKIN TUMOURS

Most benign and malignant skin tumours are more common in the elderly (Table 1). Many are related to sun exposure (p. 101). Specific disorders of photodamage include:

• *Actinic (solar) keratoses*: These are single or multiple discrete scaly hyperkeratotic rough-surfaced areas, usually less than 1cm diameter. They are seen on sun-exposed sites, especially the dorsal aspects of the hands, face and neck (Fig. 3). They are most common in those with a fair skin.

Histologically, they show hyperkeratosis, abnormal keratinocytes with loss of maturation and dermal elastosis. Actinic keratoses may regress spontaneously. However, they can progress to squamous cell carcinoma, although this is uncommon. Treatment is normally by cryosurgery, but certain lesions may be best dealt with by curettage, excision or by applying 5% 5-fluorouracil cream (Efudix) twice daily for 2–4 weeks.

A *cutaneous horn* may occasionally develop in a actinic keratoses (Fig. 4). It is treated by excision or curettage.

• *Actinic (solar) elastosis*: In solar elastosis, the sun-exposed skin is yellowed, thickened and wrinkled. On the neck, furrowed rhomboidal patterns are sometimes seen (Fig. 5) particularly in those with outside occupations such as sailors or farmers. 'Senile' comedones may develop. Thickened yellowish plaques are occasionally found.

Damaged dermal collagen with inflammation in the dermis and cartilage, is a feature of *chondrodermatitis nodularis* (p. 91 Fig. 6). Treatment is by excision.

• *Actinic cheilitis*: Excessive exposure to sun, often occupational, can induce inflammation and scaling of the lower lip. Treatment is by cryosurgery or excision.

ULCERATION

• *Leg ulcers*: Venous ulcers often start in middle age but because of their chronicity are a problem in the elderly. Ischaemic ulcers become more common with advancing years (p. 69).
• *Pressure ulcers*: A pressure ulcer starts as an area of erythema and progresses to widespread necrosis of tissue with ulceration. Deep ulcers develop over the sacrum (Fig. 7), heels, ischia and greater trochanters. Secondary infection with *Pseudomonas aeruginosa* is common.

Pressure ulcers mainly occur in the elderly who are recumbent and immobile e.g. due to a fractured femur, arthritis, unconsciousness or paraplegia. Malnutrition, reduced cutaneous sensation and atherosclerosis predispose to tissue breakdown.

Prevention is possible if at-risk patients are identified. Regular repositioning, the use of an antipressure mattress, and attention to diet and to the patient's general condition help in prevention and treatment. A necrotic eschar separates by itself in 2–4 weeks. The resulting ulcer can be covered by a semipermeable dressing e.g. Opsite. Proteolytic enzymes (Varidase) may be used to debride heel lesions. Pain relief is vital. Surgical excision and flap repair are often possible provided the patient's general condition is satisfactory.

The skin in old age

• *Asteatotic eczema* is the eczema craquelé of elderly skin. Treat with emollients and mild topical steroids.
• *Pruritus* in the elderly nearly always has a cause. Scabies, urticaria or prebullous pemphigoid are easily missed.
• *Herpes zoster* is common in old age. Aciclovir or famciclovir may make neuralgia less likely.
• *Actinic keratoses* are roughened hyperkeratotic areas in sun-exposed sites. They are often treated by cryosurgery.
• *Actinic elastosis* is a yellowed, thickened, wrinkled change in sun-exposed skin, e.g. on the neck.
• *Pressure ulcers* result from reduced sensation, immobility, malnutrition and ischaemia. Identify at-risk patients and institute means to prevent these ulcers from developing.

GENITOURINARY MEDICINE

In the UK, genitourinary medicine has traditionally been a separate speciality from dermatology, but the two are combined as 'dermatovenereology' in many countries. It has become increasingly important for those treating skin disease in Britain to know more about genitourinary disorders. Genitourinary diseases range as follows (see also Table 1):

- syphilis
- gonorrhoea
- HIV infection (p. 52)
- chlamydial infection
- pelvic inflammatory disease
- vaginitis
- chancroid
- viral warts (p. 48)
- genital herpes simplex (p. 50)
- hepatitis B and hepatitis C
- vulval/perianal dermatoses
- penile/scrotal dermatoses.

Table 1 **Other genitourinary infections**

Condition	Organisms	Clinical features	Therapy
Non-gonococcal urethritis	*Chlamydia trachomatis, Ureaplasma urealyticum*	Males: dysuria, frequency, urethral discharge	Oral doxycycline or erythromycin for 7 days
Mucopurulent cervicitis	*Chlamydia trachomatis, (Neisseria gonorrhoeae)*	Females: asymptomatic or yellow cervical exudate	Oral doxycycline or erythromycin for 7 days
Pelvic inflammatory disease	*Chlamydia trachomatis, Neisseria gonorrhoeae*	Acute abdominal pain and tenderness, fever, raised WBC	Oral doxycycline and metronidazole for 10 days
Vaginitis	*Trichomonas vaginalis, Gardnerella vaginalis,* Bacteroides, *C. albicans*	Asymptomatic or erythema, itch and discharge: male partners get urethritis and balanitis	Trichomonal/bacterial — oral metronidazole for 7 days; anticandidal topicals
Chancroid	*Haemophilus ducreyi*	Single or multiple tender, necrotic, erosive ulcers	Oral erythromycin for 7 days
Hepatitis B	Hepatitis B virus	Only 1/3–1/2 show symptoms of acute hepatitis	Vaccinate at-risk groups; interferon-alfa if chronic active

SYPHILIS (LUES)

Syphilis is a chronic infectious disease due to *Treponema pallidum*. Skin signs are seen in all three stages.

Clinical presentation

T. pallidum may rarely be acquired congenitally or from a contaminated blood transfusion, but the normal mode of transmission is through sexual intercourse.

- *Primary chancre.* About 3 weeks after sexual contact a primary chancre, a painless ulcerated button-like papule, develops at the site of inoculation. This is usually genital (Fig. 1), but oral and anal chancres are seen in homosexual males. Regional lymphadenopathy is common. Without treatment the chancre clears spontaneously in 6 weeks. Serology is not positive until 4 weeks after infection, but spirochaetes can be isolated from the chancre.
- *Secondary stage.* This phase starts 4–12 weeks after the onset of the chancre. It is characterized by a non-itchy pink or copper-coloured papular eruption on the trunk, limbs, palms and soles (p. 39). Untreated, the eruption resolves in 1-3 months. Serology is positive.
- *Tertiary stage.* About 40% of patients with untreated syphilis will develop late lesions, usually after a latent period of years. Painless nodules, sometimes with scaling, develop in annular or arcuate patterns on the face or back. Subcutaneous granulomatous gumma — usually on the face, neck or calf — ulcerate, scar and never heal completely (Fig. 2). Cardiovascular syphilis or neurosyphilis may coexist.

Management

Primary or secondary syphilis is treated with procaine penicillin, 600 mg intramuscularly daily for at least 10 days. Patients with penicillin allergy can be given erythromycin or tetracycline in appropriate dosage. Patients need contact tracing and assessment for other venereal diseases, and should be managed in a genitourinary medicine department.

GONORRHOEA

Gonorrhoea is caused by the Gram-negative diplococcus *Neisseria gonorrhoeae*. Infection may be symptomatic or asymptomatic.

Clinical presentation

Symptomatic males usually present with dysuria, frequency of micturition and a purulent urethral discharge. Females, when symptomatic, can have an abnormal vaginal discharge, dysuria, menstrual irregularity or abdominal pain. Pharyngeal and anorectal infection may produce symptoms, or may be asymptomatic. The diagnosis relies on the microscopic identification of Gram-negative intracellular diplococci from urethral (males) or endocervical (females) smears, and culture for *N. gonorrhoeae*. Serological tests are unreliable. Women with untreated gonorrhoea are at risk of developing pelvic inflammatory disease and infertility. In men, complications include urethral stricture, infertility and epididymitis.

Gonococcaemia is rare, but when observed results in fever, arthritis and pustules which are few in number and generally distributed on the hands,

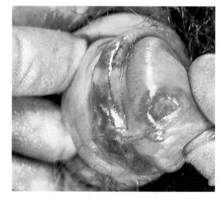

Fig. 1 **Primary chancre of syphilis.**

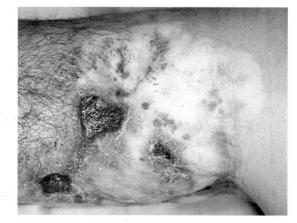

Fig. 2 **Gumma of tertiary syphilis.** The condition has caused a scarring and non-healing ulcer on the lower leg.

feet or near the large joints. This is a type of septic vasculitis which, when seen with other organisms (e.g. *N. meningitidis*), may be purpuric.

Management

Uncomplicated acute gonorrhoea should be treated with amoxycillin 2 g as a single oral dose, with probenecid 1 g orally (repeated for women). Alternatives for penicillin-sensitive patients or in the case of bacterial resistance are single doses of spectinomycin (2 g intramuscularly) or ciprofloxacin (250 mg orally or 100 mg by intravenous infusion). Pharyngeal infection may be particularly difficult to eliminate. A repeated culture to test for a cure is made 4–7 days after treatment. Patients with gonorrhoea should be screened for co-existing sexually transmitted diseases. Management is most appropriate in a department of genitourinary medicine where contact tracing can be organized.

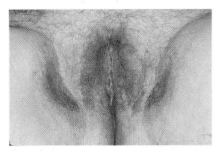

Fig. 3 **Contact dermatitis of the vulva** caused by allergy to neomycin in a cream.

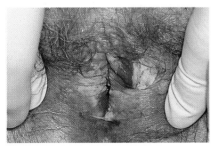

Fig. 4 **A hyperkeratotic variant of VIN.**

VULVAL DISORDERS

The vulva can be involved in many conditions and itching (pruritus vulvae), often followed by secondary lichenification, is frequent. Commonly seen dermatoses include:
- lichen sclerosus (p. 37)
- eczemas including allergic contact dermatitis (Fig. 3) and seborrhoeic dermatitis (p. 34)
- psoriasis (p. 26)
- lichen planus (p. 36)

Herpes simplex (p. 50), viral warts (p. 48), candidiasis (p. 55), venereal infections (see above) and extramammary Paget's disease (p. 84) also occur. Other specific disorders include:

- *Vulval intraepithelial neoplasia* (VIN) includes intraepidermal carcinoma and Bowenoid papulosis (Fig. 4). Cervical intraepithelial neoplasia can coexist and screening is required. Human papilloma virus infection may predispose to the precancerous change. There is a small risk of progression to invasive squamous cell carcinoma. Treatment is by cryosurgery or excision (for small areas), topical 5-fluorouracil and laser therapy. Follow up is needed.
- *Vulvodynia* is chronic vulval discomfort, often with burning and soreness. It is sometimes due to erosive vulvitis, e.g. from lichen planus or VIN. Some patients

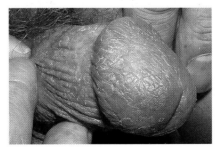

Fig. 5 **Eczema of the glans penis.**

have underlying psychological problems.
- *Genital ulceration* may occur with pemphigoid or pemphigus (p. 74), or acutely with erythema multiforme. It is also seen with Behçet's syndrome, a multisystem disorder in which recurrent oral aphthous ulceration and iridocyclitis also occur.

PENILE AND SCROTAL ERUPTIONS

Balanitis (inflammation of the penile skin: Fig. 5) and scrotal eruptions can be caused by a similar list of conditions as outlined above for vulval dermatoses. Specific disorders include:
- *Circinate balanitis*, an eroded or crusted penile eruption seen in Reiter's syndrome (p. 38)
- *Scrotal gangrene*, a necrotizing cellulitis of rapid onset, seen in diabetics. It has a mortality of 45%.

PRURITUS ANI

The perianal skin is frequently involved in infective, inflammatory and occasionally neoplastic conditions, as for the genitalia. Pruritus ani is common in middle aged men. Whatever the underlying dermatosis, faecal contamination of the perianal skin with bacteria, enzymes and allergens, causes inflammation and itch. Persistent rubbing induces lichen simplex (p. 35) or maceration, and secondary infection with bacteria or fungi. A compounding contact dermatitis due to allergy to 'over-the-counter' creams is common. Anal carcinoma, fissure or haemorrhoids, and threadworm infestation in children, should be excluded.

Treatment requires attention to personal hygiene (daily baths but avoid of soap) and topical use of an emollient, antiseptic or steroid preparation.

Genitourinary medicine

Syphilis
- The primary chancre appears 3 weeks after sexual contact.
- The papular non-pruritic eruption of the secondary stage is seen 4–12 weeks following the chancre.
- Tertiary syphilis may be delayed several years.
- Treatment is with procaine penicillin.

Gonorrhoea
- Males present with dysuria, frequency and a urethral discharge.
- Females complain of a vaginal discharge, dysuria and abdominal pain.
- Infection may be asymptomatic.
- Late sequelae include pelvic inflammatory disease and infertility.
- Treatment is with amoxycillin or spectinomycin.

Vulval disorders
- Common vulval disorders include lichen sclerosus, eczemas, psoriasis and vulvodynia.
- Vulval intraepithelial neoplasia requires long term follow-up and cervical screening.
- Chronic ulceration may indicate a blistering disorder or Behçet's syndrome.
- Secondary contact dermatitis due to medicament allergy is common.

Pruritus ani
- Is common in middle aged men.
- May be due to the irritant effects of faecal contamination on perianal skin.
- Anal carcinoma, fissure and haemorrhoids must be excluded.
- Local hygiene measures and a topical antiseptic or steroid are prescribed.
- Secondary allergic contact dermatitis is common.

RACIALLY PIGMENTED SKIN

Common dermatoses may show variable manifestations in different races due to differences in pigmentation, hair or the response of skin to external stimuli. In addition, some conditions have a distinct racial predisposition. The response of darkly pigmented skin to injury and to certain therapeutic modalities needs to be taken into account when planning a programme of management.

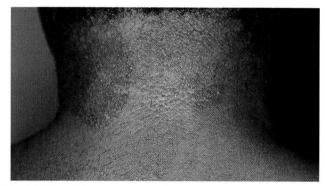

Fig. 1 **Lichen simplex chronicus showing hyperpigmentation and lichenification.**

DEFINITION OF RACE

The characteristics of our species *Homo sapiens* are continuously variable, and hence the division into 'races' is — to some extent — artificial. However, there are obvious differences between groups of humans, and these differences have an influence on the appearance of and susceptibility to disease. Most definitions of a '*race*' are unsatisfactory, but perhaps the best is 'a population which differs significantly from other populations in regard to the frequency of one or more of the genes that it possesses.' Obviously this definition allows even rather small groups to be classified as a race!

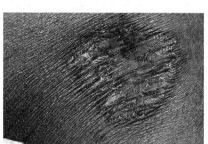

Fig. 2 **Lichen planus with hyperpigmentation.**

It is generally assumed that changes in gene frequency result from mutation, natural selection and 'accidental' loss. Some changes are thought to be the result of adaptation to environmental conditions, although it is not always obvious what advantage is conferred. Racial classification has relied on physical characteristics, often skeletal, although hair form and skin colour are taken into account. The main divisions are:

- *Australoid*: e.g. Australian aborigines
- *Capoid*: e.g. bushmen, hottentots
- *Caucasoid*: Europeans, people of the Mediterranean, Middle East and most of the Indian subcontinent
- *Mongoloid*: peoples of East Asia, Eskimos, American indians
- *Negroid*: e.g. Black Africans.

RACIAL DIFFERENCES IN NORMAL SKIN

The most obvious difference is in pigmentation (p. 7), but hair forms and colour also vary. Mongoloid hair is straight and has the largest diameter, African hair is short, spiralled, drier and more brittle than that of other races, and caucasoid hair may be wavy, straight or helical. Hair colour is predominantly black in mongoloids and Africans, and black, blond or red in caucasoids. Body hair is most profuse in caucasoids. The African stratum corneum differs from the caucasoid by showing greater intercellular adhesion and a higher lipid content.

DISEASES THAT SHOW RACIALLY DEPENDENT VARIATIONS

In pigmented skin, eruptions that in white caucasoid skin appear red or brown may be black, grey or purple, and pigmentation can mask an erythematous reaction. Inflammation in pigmented skin often provokes a hyperpigmentary (Figs 1 & 2), or hypopigmentary reaction (Table 1). Follicular, papular and annular patterns are more common in pigmented skin than in caucasoid. In addition, some skin disorders show an inter-racial variation in prevalence (Table 2).

Table 1 **Causes of hypopigmentation in a pigmented skin**

Division	Disorder
Infections	Leprosy, pinta, pityriasis versicolor
Papulosquamous disorders	Pityriasis rosea/alba, psoriasis (occasionally), seborrhoeic dermatitis
Physical/chemical agents	Burns, cryotherapy, hydroquinone, topical potent steroids
Post-inflammatory	Discoid LE, systemic sclerosis, sarcoidosis
Other	Vitiligo

Table 2 **Diseases with racially-dependent variations**

Skin disorder	Caucasoid	Mongoloid	Black African
Acne	Most severe	Least common	Hyperpigmented lesions
Atopic eczema	Most common with Western lifestyle	Lichenification is seen	Follicular and hyperpigmented lesions are found
Keloid	May occur	More frequent	More frequent
Lichen planus	Can show some pigmentation	Often hyperpigmented	Often hyperpigmented
Melanocytic naevi	Very common	A few may be present	Uncommon
Psoriasis	Common (2% prevalence)	Rare (0.3% prevalence but increasing)	East > West Africans: plaques bluish, leave pigmentation
Sarcoidosis	Less common	Less common	In US, ten times more common than in caucasoids
Skin cancer	Most common in Northern Europeans	Intermediate prevalence	Uncommon
Vitiligo	Same prevalence, least obvious	Same prevalence, more obvious	Same prevalence, most obvious

DISEASES WITH A DISTINCT RACIAL OR ETHNIC PREDISPOSITION

Hair disorders

Racially-dependent hair conditions are most common in black Africans and include the following:

- *Folliculitis keloidalis* describes discrete follicular papules, often keloids, at the back of the neck in African males (Fig. 3). Intralesional steroids may help.
- *Pseudofolliculitis barbae* is a common disorder in African males and is characterized by inflammatory papules and pustules in the beard area. It is thought to result from hairs growing back into the skin (Fig. 4). Treatment is difficult but includes attention to shaving technique and the topical use of antibiotics and steroids.
- *Traction alopecia* is mainly seen in Africans because of the practice of plaiting or tightly braiding the hair (Fig. 5). Hairs are loosened from their follicles. The temples are often affected.
- *Hot-comb alopecia* is a traction alopecia caused by applying a hot comb to oiled hair in order to straighten it (curly African hair is usually straightened by chemical methods).

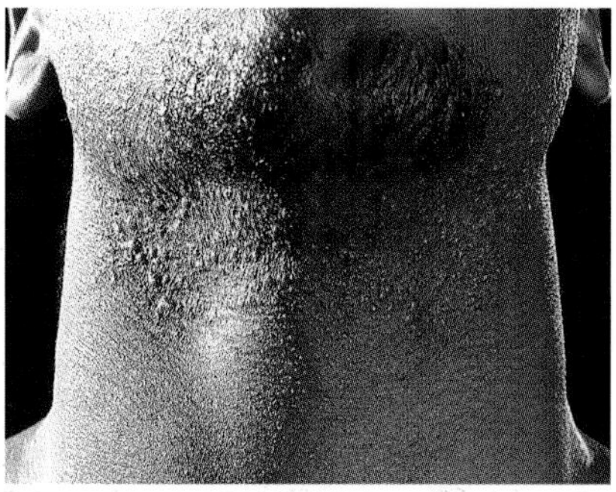

Pigmentary changes

Pigmentary abnormalities, both as variation of 'normal' and otherwise, are also common. These include the following:

- *Dermatosis papulosa nigra* describes small, seborrhoeic wart-like papules often seen on the face in black Africans.
- *Lines of hypo- or hyper-pigmentation*, often on the upper arms, are not infrequently found in black Africans.
- *Longitudinal nail pigmentation* and macular pigmentation of the palms and soles also occur mainly in negroids.
- *Mongolian spot* is a slate-brown pigmentation at the sacral area in a baby and is found in 100% of mongoloids, 70% or more of Africans and 10% of caucasoids. It usually fades by the age of 6 years.

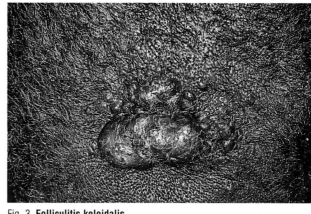

Fig. 3 **Folliculitis keloidalis.**

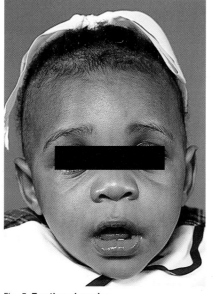

Fig. 4 **Pseudofolliculitis barbae.**

Fig. 5 **Traction alopecia.**

- *Naevus of Ota* is a macular, slate-grey pigmentation in the upper trigeminal area which may involve the sclera (Fig. 6). It is seen most frequently in mongoloids.

Other conditions

A racial preponderance is also seen with the following conditions.

- *Sickle cell disease* occurs in Africans. The main cutaneous findings are painful oedema of the hands and feet, caused by infarction in the small bones, and leg ulceration.
- *Vascular naevi*, such as the port-wine stain naevus, are more common in caucasoids than in other races.

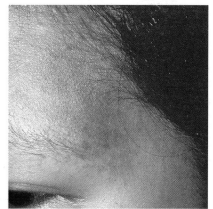

Fig. 6 **Naevus of Ota.**

Racially pigmented skin

- *A race* is a genetically defined group, although the characteristics of *H. sapiens* are continuously variable.
- *The most numerous races* are mongoloids, black Africans and caucasoids.
- Eruptions that appear red or brown in caucasoids may be *black*, *grey* or *purple* in those with pigmented skin.
- Inflammatory dermatoses tend to become *lichenified* in mongoloids and may be *follicular* in black Africans.
- Skin trauma (e.g. burns or from cryotherapy), topical steroids and some dermatoses may cause *hypopigmentation* in pigmented skin.
- *Hair disorders*, e.g. pseudofolliculitis, keloidal change or traction alopecia, are common in black Africans.
- *Pigmentary lines* are frequently found on the limbs or nails in black Africans and other races.
- *Sacral mongolian spots* are found in most mongoloid and black African babies but in only a few caucasoid infants.
- *Vascular and melanocytic naevi* are more common in caucasoids than in other races.

OCCUPATION AND THE SKIN

Skin disorders make up 60% of all reported occupational disease and are responsible for much lost productivity. An occupational dermatosis is defined as a skin condition that is primarily caused by components of the work environment and which would not have occurred unless the individual were doing that job.

DIAGNOSIS

Proving a work association can be difficult. The following give clues:

- contact with a known noxious agent
- similar skin disease in other workers
- consistent exposure-to-onset time course
- attacks appear with exposure, improve on withdrawal
- site and type of eruption consistent with exposure
- corroboration by patch testing

Table 1 **Rarer occupational skin disorders**

Condition	Presentation	Occupational exposure
Argyria (Fig. 4)	Slate grey pigmentation on face, hands, sclerae	Industrial processes e.g. silver smelters
Chloracne (Fig. 5)	Multiple open and closed comedones on cheeks and behind ears	Halogenated aromatic hydrocarbons e.g. contamination during manufacture
Occupational vitiligo (p. 70)	Symmetrical pigment loss on face and hands	Substituted phenols or catechols in oils, at coking plant
Tar keratoses (Fig. 6)	Small keratotic warts on face/hand, premalignant	Tar and pitch, e.g. road work or coking plant: UV is co-carcinogen
Vibration white finger	Blanching and pain in digits, later swelling and impaired fine movement	Hand-held vibrating tools e.g. rock drillers, chainsaw operators

Contact dermatitis is the commonest work-related skin disease and is more often irritant than allergic. Contact urticaria is being increasingly recognised. Other occupational dermatoses are listed in Table 1. Certain infections, e.g. anthrax (p. 47), orf (p. 49) and tinea corporis (p. 54) may be occupational. Heat, cold, ultraviolet radiation and X-rays can cause industrial disease.

CONTACT DERMATITIS

It is often difficult to differentiate between allergic and irritant causes.

AETIOPATHOGENESIS

Many industrial substances are irritants and some are also allergens (p. 31). Water, detergents, alkalis, coolant oils and solvents are important irritants. Common allergens include chromate, rubber chemicals, preservatives, nickel, fragrances, epoxy resins and phenol-formaldehyde resins (Table 2).

Irritant dermatitis frequently results from cumulative exposure to multiple types of irritant. Because an irritant dermatitis increases epidermal penetration by allergens it predisposes to superimposed contact sensitization. Similarly, allergic contact dermatitis renders skin vulnerable to attack by irritants.

Constitutional factors, especially atopic eczema, predispose to contact dermatitis. Environmental factors such as friction, occlusion, heat, cold, dry air from air conditioning, or sudden swings in air temperature or humidity also have an effect.

CLINICAL PRESENTATION

The hands are affected, alone or with other sites, in 80–90% of occupational cases. The arms can be involved if not covered and the face and neck are affected if there is exposure to dust or

Table 2 **Contact dermatitis hazards in selected occupations**

Occupation	Irritants	Allergens
Bakers	Flour, detergent, sugar, enzymes	Flavouring, oil, antitoxidant
Building trade workers	Cement, glass wool, acid, preservatives	Cement (Cr, Co), rubber, resin, wood
Caterers, cooks	Meat, fish, fruit, veg, detergent	Veg/fruit, cutlery (Ni), rubber glove, spice
Cleaners	Detergent, solvent	Rubber glove, nickel, fragrance
Dental personnel	Detergent, soap, acrylate, flux	Rubber, acrylate, fragrance, mercury
Electronics assemblers	Solder, solvent, fibreglass, acid	Cr, Co, Ni, acrylate, epoxy resin
Hairdressers	Shampoo, bleach, perm lotion, soap	Dye, rubber, fragrance, Ni, thioglycolate
Metal workers	Cutting oils, cleanser, solvent	Preservative, Ni, Cr, Co, antioxidant
Office workers	Paper, fibreglass, dry atmosphere	Rubber, Ni, dye, glue, copying paper
Textile workers	Solvent, bleach, fibre, formaldehyde	Formaldehyde resin, dye, Ni
Veterinarians, farmers	Disinfectant, animal secretion	Rubber, antibiotics, plants, preservative

Case history 1: Contact dermatitis

A 17-year-old girl who had had childhood atopic eczema started as a hairdressing apprentice. Within 8 weeks she developed a hand dermatitis (Fig. 1) unresponsive to emollients and topical steroids. Patch testing was positive for ammonium thioglycolate (a permanent-wave agent) and nickel. A diagnostic was made of contact dermatitis with irritant and allergic

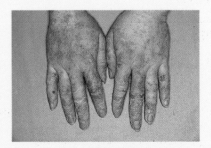

Fig. 1 **Hand dermatitis in a hairdresser.**

components, in an individual with underlying endogenous eczema. Her dermatitis cleared within weeks when she left hairdressing to work in an office.

fumes. Cement workers often have lower leg and foot dermatitis in addition to hand changes. Allergy to rubber chemicals can cause a dermatitis from rubber gloves or boots. Some workers develop 'hardening', an adaptive tolerance to irritants or allergies.

Occupational dermatitis appears at any age but peaks at each end of working life. In bakers and hairdressers, dermatitis appears early. In cement workers, chromate dermatitis requires a few years to develop. Cumulative irritant dermatitis appears after several years exposure.

DIFFERENTIAL DIAGNOSIS

Contact dermatitis due to non-occupational exposure and endogenous eczemas need considering. Often occupational dermatitis is multifactorial, with irritants, allergens, endogenous factors and secondary bacterial infection all causally involved.

MANAGEMENT

Patch testing (p. 118) is required if there is exposure to known allergens. A factory visit helps to ascertain the exact nature of irritant or allergen exposure.

Case history 2: Chromate dermatitis

A 30-year-old man had been employed for 3 years making pipes out of cement. This involved exposure to wet cement, despite him wearing gloves and overalls. He developed a dermatitis on the hands (Fig. 2), arms and lower legs. Patch testing showed chromate allergy. He received compensation for having an industrial disease but despite changing his occupation to driving, he continued to have hand dermatitis.

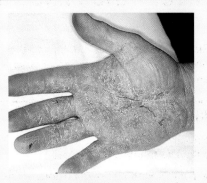

Fig. 2 **Hand dermatitis in a cement worker.**

Once recognised, occupational exposure to a causative agent can be minimised but this does not always produce an improvement. Chromate allergy is particularly intransigent. Any dermatitis is treated along standard lines with special attention to hand care. Barrier creams are of dubious value.

CONTACT URTICARIA

Some proteins and chemicals provoke immediate urticaria (p. 103). The release of mast cell histamine or other mediators may or may not be IgE-mediated. Pruritus, erythema and whealing appear within minutes and last a few hours.

Occupational contacts include latex in rubber gloves, foods (e.g. fish, potato, eggs, flour, spices, meats and numerous fruits), balsam of Peru (a perfume and flavouring agent) and animal saliva. Contact dermatitis may coexist.

Latex contact urticaria is a problem in healthcare workers. Anaphylaxis may occur if there is a massive latex exposure e.g. in a patient exposed to surgeon's gloves during abdominal surgery.

Case history 3: Contact urticaria

A 40-year-old female nurse gave a 12 month history of itching, swelling and redness on her hands (Fig. 3) which developed within minutes of wearing disposable latex gloves. Patch testing was negative but a prick test was positive for latex (confirmed by specific IgE test). Her symptoms resolved when she changed to polyvinyl chloride gloves.

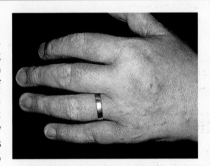

Fig. 3 **Contact urticaria in a nurse.**

PREVENTION

Reducing the contact time between the skin and noxious substances is the aim. It is achieved by:

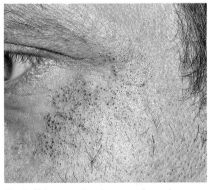

Fig. 5 **Chloracne showing comedones in a man exposed to dioxin contaminants.**

- improved work practices, e.g. increased automation
- substituting an alternative, e.g. PVC instead of rubber
- provision of protective clothing
- taking better care of the skin

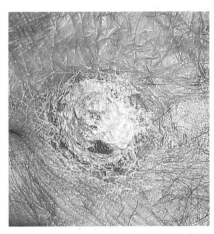

Fig. 6 **A tar keratosis in a coking plant worker.**

Recognising an occupational disease may highlight faulty work practices which can be corrected. Compensation may be due.

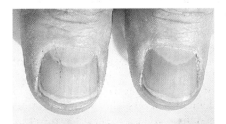

Fig. 4 **Blue discoloration of the nails in a silver smelter with argyria.**

Occupation and the skin

- *Occurrence:* industrial skin disease is common, especially contact dermatitis.
- *Causation:* occupational contact dermatitis is caused more by irritants than allergens but often is multifactorial.
- *Predisposition:* previous atopic eczema predisposes to occupational contact dermatitis.
- *Patch testing:* can help identify an allergen, e.g. chromate or rubber chemicals
- *Contact urticaria* to latex is increasing in healthcare workers.
- *Prevention:* occupational skin disease is minimized by reducing the contact time of noxious agents with the skin and by increasing awareness of the problem.

IMMUNOLOGICAL TESTS

Clinical and laboratory tests of an immunological nature are valuable in the diagnosis and management of certain skin diseases. Patch tests are helpful in the investigation of *contact dermatitis*, prick tests are sometimes of use in *atopic disease*, and immunofluorescent studies on biopsied skin (or on serum) are essential in the diagnosis of *bullous disorders* and in some other conditions such as connective tissue diseases (e.g. lupus erythematosus) or vasculitis.

PRICK TESTS

Prick testing detects *immediate (type I) hypersensitivity* and is mediated by the antigen-triggered IgE-mediated release of vasoactive substances from skin mast cells (p. 11). Small drops of commercially prepared antigen solutions are placed on marked areas on the forearm and pricked into the skin using separate sterile no. 26G ('brown') needles. The epidermis is punctured by gently pressing the needle, bevel edge down, in a horizontal manner onto the skin surface through the test solution. The sites are inspected at 15 minutes and a positive result is regarded, by convention, as one showing a wheal of 4mm or greater (Fig. 1). Patients should have stopped antihistamines 48 hours before the test. Prick tests are used, in atopic subjects, to demonstrate allergy to inhalants (e.g. house dust mite) or to foods (e.g. hen's egg or peanuts), and are positive in

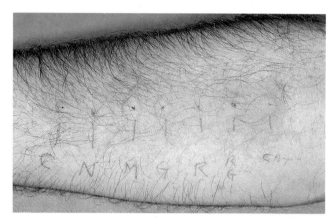

Fig. 1 **Positive prick tests in an atopic subject.**

patients with contact urticaria to latex (p. 117). A positive test correlates well with a positive radioallergosorbent test (RAST), which detects allergen-specific IgE. The risk of anaphylaxis is very small, but resuscitation facilities, including adrenaline for intramuscular injection and oxygen, are mandatory.

PATCH TESTING

The epicutaneous patch test detects *cell-mediated (type IV) hypersensitivity* (p. 11) and is very helpful in the investigation of contact dermatitis. Commercially prepared allergens are available in the correct concentration for testing, usually in petrolatum as a base. The procedure is shown in Figure 2.

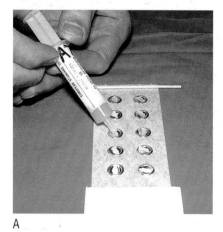

A

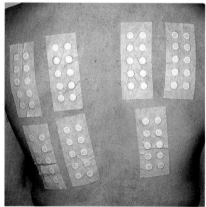

B

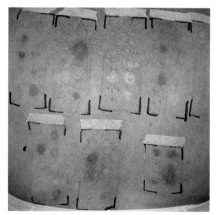

C

Fig. 2 **Patch testing methodology**

A Patch tests are prepared
Small amounts of test substances are applied to the small aluminium discs on adhesive tape (Finn chambers) that are used for patch testing. The exact range of test substances selected depends on the clinical problem, the site of the dermatitis, the environmental contacts and the patient's occupation.

B Patch tests are applied
A 'standard battery' of 23 substances is applied to every patient, with additional allergens as necessary. A record sheet is

kept. The patches are fixed to the upper back, left on for 2 days and then removed after marking the top margin of each test strip with adhesive tape.

C Patch tests are read
Numerous *allergic-positive patch test sites* are shown. A positive allergic response is manifest by a localized eczema reaction which is scored according to the following convention:

+/−   doubtful: faint erythema only
+   weak: erythema, maybe papules
++   strong: vesicles, infiltration

+++   extreme: bullous
IR   irritant (of various types, but often showing a glazed circumscribed area, frequently with increased skin markings).

The test sites are read for a second time at 4 days, since not uncommonly a positive reaction does not appear until this time. The results are interpreted in the light of the clinical situation: a positive reaction is not always relevant to the current skin problem. Common allergens and their sources are shown on page 31.

IMMUNOFLUORESCENCE

Immunofluorescence, either direct (on the patient's skin) or indirect (using the patient's serum reacted with an animal substrate) (Fig. 3), is helpful in making a diagnosis in the *autoimmune blistering diseases* (Table 1). Bullous disorders such as pemphigoid (Fig. 4) and pemphigus (Fig. 5) (p. 74) are characterized by the deposition of organ-specific autoantibodies (usually IgG) in the skin and, less easily demonstrated, by the presence of these autoantibodies in the serum. Dermatitis herpetiformis (Fig. 6) and other conditions such as leucocytoclastic vasculitis or lupus erythematosus often show the deposition of immunoglobulin or complement components in the patient's skin.

Table 1 Immunofluorescence in bullous disease

Bullous disorder	Direct immuno-fluorescence (skin)	Indirect immuno-fluorescence (serum)
Bullous pemphigoid	Linear IgG/C3 at BMZ in 80% (IgA/IgM in 25%)	Linear IgG at BMZ in 75%
Pemphigus vulgaris	Intercellular epidermal IgG/C3 in 100% (IgA/IgM in 20%)	Intercellular IgG in 90% (the antibody titre reflects disease activity)
Dermatitis herpetiformis	Granular IgA deposition at dermal papilla (100%)	Absent
Linear IgA disease	Linear IgA at BMZ in 80% (IgG/IgM/C3 in 10%)	Linear IgA at BMZ found in some cases

Fig. 3 **Immunofluorescence.** In *direct immunofluorescence*, usually done on peri-lesional skin, the antibodies or complement components are detected by reacting the freshly-cut skin sections with an antibody directed against the specific immunoglobulin or complement fraction and labelled with a marker (usually fluorescein) which shows up when the section is examined under ultra-violet radiation. The *indirect method* is a two-step procedure that involves the use of cut sections of an animal substrate (e.g. monkey oesophagus). The patient's diluted serum (containing the putative antibody) is placed on this section, incubated for an hour or so and then revealed using a fluorescein-tagged anti-human immunoglobulin antibody which is demonstrated by examining with ultraviolet radiation.

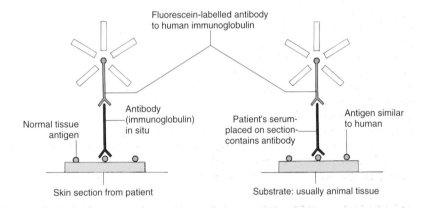

Direct immunofluorescence   **Indirect immunofluorescence**

Fluorescein-labelled antibody to human immunoglobulin

Normal tissue antigen — Antibody (immunoglobulin) in situ

Skin section from patient

Patient's serum placed on section contains antibody — Antigen similar to human

Substrate: usually animal tissue

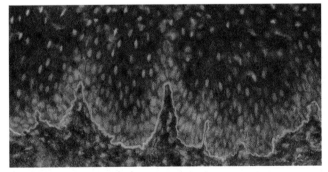

Fig. 4 **Bullous pemphigoid.** Indirect immunofluorescence demonstrates a linear band of IgG antibodies along the basement membrane zone (BMZ) using monkey oesophagus as substrate. These antibodies are directed against bullous pemphigoid antigens, which are located in the lamina lucida and synthesized by the basal keratinocytes. BP antigens have molecular weights of 230 and 180 kDa.

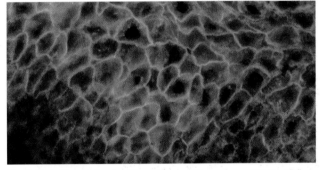

Fig. 5 **Pemphigus vulgaris.** Direct immunofluorescence shows IgG antibodies, directed against the transmembrane glycoprotein desmoglein (MW 130 kDa), in a chicken-wire pattern throughout the epidermis.

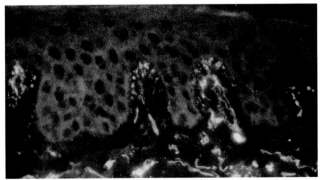

Fig. 6 **Dermatitis herpetiformis.** Direct immunofluorescence reveals the deposition of IgA in a granular pattern at the dermal papillae. This is diagnostic for dermatitis herpetiformis (p. 75) although it is unlikely that the eruption is solely due to the presence of this IgA.

Immunological tests

- *Prick tests* detect type I (IgE-mediated) hypersensitivity and demonstrate inhalant and food allergies.
- *Patch tests* detect type IV (cell-mediated) hypersensitivity and are helpful in investigating contact dermatitis.
- *Direct immunofluorescence* detects immunoglobulin and complement deposition in the skin and is very useful in the diagnosis of bullous disorders.
- *Indirect immunofluorescence* uses an animal substrate to detect antibodies in a patient's serum. It is often positive in pemphigus and pemphigoid, and sometimes in linear IgA disease, but is negative in dermatitis herpetiformis.

BIBLIOGRAPHY

Microanatomy, derivatives, physiology and biochemistry of the skin

Bannister L H 1995 *Integumental system*. In: Williams P L, Bannister L H, Berry M M et al (eds) *Gray's Anatomy* 38th edn. Churchill Livingstone, Edinburgh pp 375–424

Ebling F J G 1992 *Functions of the skin*. In: Champion R H, Burton J L, Ebling F J G (eds) *Textbook of Dermatology* 5th edn. Blackwell Science, Oxford, pp 125–55

Immunology of the skin

Roitt I, Brostoff J, Male D 1996 *Immunology* 4th edn. Mosby, London

Molecular genetics and the skin

Mueller R F, Young I D 1995 *Emery's Elements of Medical Genetics* 9th edn. Churchill Livingstone, Edinburgh

Terminology of skin lesions, taking a history and examining the skin

Lawrence C M, Cox N H 1993 *Physical Signs in Dermatology*. Mosby Yearbook, London

Champion R H, Burton J L 1992 *Diagnosis of skin disease*. In: Champion R H, Burton J L, Ebling F J G (eds) *Textbook of Dermatology* 5th edn. Blackwell Science, Oxford pp 157–70

Basics of medical therapy

Arndt K A 1995 *Manual of Dermatologic Therapeutics* 2nd edn. Little Brown & Co, Boston

Epidemiology of skin disease

Barker D J P, Rose G 1990 *Epidemiology in Medical Practice* 4th edn. Churchill Livingstone, Edinburgh

Body image, the psyche and the skin

Cotterill J A 1983 *Psychodermatology* Semin Dermatol 2: 171–226

Psoriasis

Zachariae H 1990 *Management of severe psoriasis*. In: Champion R H, Pye R J (eds) *Recent Advances in Dermatology 8*. Churchill Livingstone, Edinburgh 1–20

van de Kerkhof P C M, Mier P D 1986 *Textbook of Psoriasis*. Churchill Livingstone, Edinburgh

The eczemas

Ruzicka T, Ring J, Przybilla B (eds) 1991 *Handbook of Atopic Eczema*. Springer-Verlag, Berlin

Rycroft R J G, Menné T, Frosch P J (eds) 1995 *Textbook of Contact Dermatitis* 2nd edn. Springer-Verlag, Berlin

Lichenoid eruptions

Boyd A S, Neldner K H 1991 *Lichen planus*. J Am Acad Dermatol 25: 593–619

Papulosquamous eruptions

Parsons J M 1986 *Pityriasis rosea: update*. J Am Acad Dermatol 15: 159–67

Erythroderma

Weiselthier J S, Koh H K 1990 *Sézary syndrome: diagnosis, prognosis and critical review of treatment options*. J Am Acad Dermatol 22: 381–401

Cohen P R, Prystowsky J H 1989 *Pityriasis rubra pilaris: a review of diagnosis and treatment*. J Am Acad Dermatol 20: 801–7

Photodermatology

Norris P G 1993 *Light sensitivity*. Hospital Update, August: 438–42

Bacterial, viral and fungal infections

Bisno A L, Stevens D L 1996 *Streptococcal infections of skin and soft tissue*. N Engl J Med 334: 240–5

Sanders C D, Nesbitt L T 1995 *The Skin in Infections*. Williams and Wilkins, Baltimore

Crissey J T, Lang H, Parish L D (eds) 1994 *Manual of Medical Mycology*. Blackwell Science, Oxford

HIV disease and immunodeficiency syndromes

Leigh I M, Glover M T 1995 *Cutaneous warts and tumours in immunosuppressed patients*. J Roy Soc Med 88: 61–2

Penneys N 1995 *Skin Manifestations of AIDS* 2nd edn. Martin Dunitz, London

Tropical infections and infestations

Lockwood D N, Pasvol G 1994 *Recent advances in tropical medicine*. Br Med J 308: 1559–62

Schaller K 1994 *Colour Atlas of Tropical Dermatology and Venereology*. Springer-Verlag, Berlin

Infestations

Alexander J O'D 1984 *Arthropods and Human Skin*. Springer-Verlag, Berlin

Sebaceous and sweat gland disorders

Cunliffe W J 1989 *Acne*. Martin Dunitz, London

Disorders of hair

Olsen E A (ed.) 1994 *Disorders of Hair Growth: Diagnosis and Treatment*. McGraw-Hill, New York

Disorders of nails

de Berker D A R, Baran R, Dawber R P R 1995 *Handbook of Diseases of the Nails and their Management*. Blackwell Science, Oxford

Vascular and lymphatic diseases and leg ulcers

Mortimer P S 1990 *Lymphatics*. In: Champion R H, Pye R J (eds) *Recent Advances in Dermatology 8*. Churchill Livingstone, Edinburgh 175–92

Falanga V, Eaglstein W H 1995 *Leg and Foot Ulcers: a Clinician's Guide.* Martin Dunitz, London

Pigmentation

Gawkrodger D J *Vitiligo.* In: Weetman A P (ed.) *Endocrine Autoimmunity and Associated Conditions.* Kluwer Academic, Dordrecht, in press

Castenet J, Frenck E, Graupe K et al 1995 *Melasma: New Approaches to Treatment.* Martin Dunitz, London

Urticaria and angioedema

Grattan C E H 1994 *The urticarias.* In: Lawson D H, Toft A D (eds*) Current Medicine 4.* Churchill Livingstone, Edinburgh 83–96

Blistering disorders

Graham-Brown R A C, Monk B E 1988 *Blistering eruptions.* In: Monk B E, Graham-Brown R A C, Sarkany I (eds) *Skin Disorders in the Elderly.* Blackwell Science, Oxford 113–32

Connective tissue diseases

Venables P J W 1993 *Diagnosis and treatment of systemic lupus erythematosus.* Br Med J 307: 663–6

Perez M I, Kohn S R 1993 *Systemic sclerosis.* J Am Acad Dermatol 28: 525–47

Vasculitis and the reactive erythemas

Jorizzo J L 1993 *Classification of vasculitis.* J Invest Dermatol 100: 106S–10S

Skin changes in internal medicine

Callen J P, Jorizzo J L, Greer K E et al (eds) 1995 *Dermatological Signs of Internal Disease* 2nd edn. W B Saunders, Philadelphia

Drug eruptions

Breathnach S M, Hintner H 1992 *Adverse Drug Reactions and the Skin.* Blackwell Science, Oxford

Associations with malignancy

Gawkrodger D J 1991 *Cutaneous manifestations of malignant disease.* Current Practice in Surgery 3: 212–7

Inherited keratinization, blistering, neurocutaneous and other syndromes

Moss C, Savin J 1995 *Dermatology and the New Genetics.* Blackwell Science, Oxford

Harper J I (ed.) 1996 *Inherited Skin Disorders.* Butterworth Heinemann, Oxford

Benign tumours and naevi

DeCoste S D, Stern R S 1993 *Diagnosis and treatment of nevomelanocytic lesions of the skin.* Arch Dermatol 129: 57–62

McGibbon D H 1988 *Skin tumours.* In: Monk B E, Graham-Brown R A C, Sarkany I, (eds) *Skin Disorders in the Elderly.* Blackwell Science, Oxford 181–204

Malignant melanoma

Kirkham N, Cotton D W K, Lallemand K C et al (eds) 1992 *Diagnosis and Management of Melanoma in Clinical Practice.* Springer-Verlag, London

Malignant epidermal and dermal tumours and premalignant epidermal disorders

MacKie R M 1995 *Skin Cancer* 2nd edn. Martin Dunitz, London

Ultraviolet radiation and the skin

Marks R 1995 *Sun and the Skin.* Martin Dunitz, London

British Photodermatology Group 1993 *Guidelines for PUVA.* Br J Dermatol 130: 246–55

The skin in old age

Marks R *Skin Disease in Old Age* 2nd edn. Martin Dunitz, London, in press

Monk B E, Graham-Brown R A C, Sarkany I (eds) 1988 *Skin Disorders in the Elderly.* Blackwell Science, Oxford

Cosmetics

Baran R, Maibach H I (eds) 1994 *Cosmetic Dermatology.* Martin Dunitz, London

Basic dermatological surgery

Burge S, Colver G, Lester R 1996 *Simple Skin Surgery* 2nd edn. Blackwell Science, Oxford

Dawber R, Colver G, Jackson A 1997 *Cutaneous Cryosurgery: Principles and Clinical Practice* 2nd edn. Martin Dunitz, London

New trends in dermatological treatment

Sober A J, Fitzpatrick T B (eds) *1995 Year Book of Dermatology* Mosby Yearbook, St Louis 157–74

Maddin S (ed.) 1991 *Current Dermatologic Therapy* 2nd edn. W B Saunders, Philadelphia

Paediatric dermatology

Harper J 1990 *Handbook of Paediatric Dermatology* 2nd edn. Butterworth, London

Verbov J L 1988 *Essential Paediatric Dermatology.* Clinical Press, Bristol

Genitourinary medicine

Lynch P J, Edwards L 1994 *Genital Dermatology.* Churchill Livingstone, New York

Racially pigmented skin

Archer C B, Robertson S J 1995 *Black and White Skin Diseases: an Atlas and Text.* Blackwell Science, Oxford

Occupation and the skin

Adams R M 1990 *Occupational Skin Disease* 2nd edn. Grune and Stratton, New York

Immunological tests

Dahl M V 1996 *Clinical Immunodermatology* 3rd edn. Mosby Yearbook, St Louis

SELF-HELP GROUPS

Patients with skin disease, especially those with a chronic condition, often find it helpful to meet and speak to others with the same problem. *Patient help groups* fulfil a particular need by helping the patient to come to terms with his or her condition, by informing the patient through meetings and publications of advances in treatments and benefits which may be available to them, and by providing support through difficult times. Several of them are also actively engaged in fundraising to support research and are involved in advancing their cause, and that of dermatology generally, in the local and national media. The addresses of some of the patient help groups, and of other organizations that are of service to those with skin problems, are given below.

ADDRESSES IN THE UNITED KINGDOM

Acne Support Group
PO Box 230
Hayes NB4 0UT

Albino Fellowship
16 Neward Crescent
Prestwick KA9 2JB

British Association of Cancer United Patients (BACUP)
3 Bath Place
London EC2A 3JR

British Association of Dermatologists
19 Fitzroy Square
London W1P 5PQ

British Red Cross
(provide a camouflage cosmetic service)
9 Grosvenor Crescent
London SW1X 7EJ

Changing Faces
(for patients with facial disfigurement)
27 Cowper Street
London EC2A 4AP

Coeliac Society,
(for dermatitis herpetiformis patients on a gluten-free diet)
PO Box 181
London NW2 2QY

Dystrophic Epidermolysis Bullosa Research Association (DEBRA)
12 Wellington Business Park
Crowthorne
Berkshire RG11 6LS

Hairline International
1668 High Street
Knowle B93 0LY

In Touch Trust
(Group for rare problems in children)
10 Norman Road
Sale
Cheshire M33 3DF

L.E.P.R.A. (Leprosy)
Fairfax House
Causton Road
Colchester CO1 1PU

Lupus UK
51 North Street
Romford RM1 1BW

Naevus Support Group
58 Necton Road
Wheathampstead
Hertfordshire AL4 8AU

National Eczema Society
163 Eversholt Street
London NW1 1BU

National Self-Help Centre (NCV)
8 All Saints Street
London N1 9RL

Neurofibromatosis Association
82 London Road
Kingston-upon-Thames KT2 6PX

Psoriasis Association
7 Milton Street
Northampton NN2 7JG

Raynaud's and Scleroderma Association Trust
112 Crewe Road
Alsager
Cheshire ST7 2JA

Scleroderma Society
61 Sandpit Lane
St Albans
Hertfordshire AL1 4EY

Terence Higgins Trust Ltd.
52–54 Grey's Inn Road
WC1X 8JN

Tuberous Sclerosis Association of Great Britain
Little Barnsley Farm
Catshill
Bromsgrove B61 0NQ

Vitiligo Society
19 Fitzroy Square
London W1P 5PQ

ADDRESSES IN THE UNITED STATES

American Academy of Dermatology
930 N. Meacham Road
Schaumberg IL 60173-4965

American Cancer Society
1599 Clifton Road NE
Atlanta, GA 30329

American Hair Loss Council
100 Independence Place, Suite 315A
Tyler, TX 75703

Dystrophic Epidermolysis Bullosa Research Association (DEBRA)
141 Fifth Avenue, Suite 7S
New York, NY 10010

Eczema Association for Science and Education
1221 SW Yarnhill, Suite 303
Portland, OR 97205

Lupus Foundation of America
4 Research Place, Sceite 180
Rockville, MO 20850-3226

National Alopecia Areata Foundation
710 'C' Street, Suite11
San Rafael, California 94901-0760

National Neurofibromatosis Foundation Inc
95 Pine Street, 16th Floor
New York, NY 10005

National Psoriasis Foundation
6600 SW 92nd, Suite 300
Portland, OR 97223

National Tuberous Sclerosis Association Inc
8000 Corporate Drive, Suite 120
Landover, MD 20785

National Vitiligo Foundation Inc
PO Box 6337
Tyler, TX 75711

Skin Cancer Foundation
245 Fifth Avenue, Suite 2402
New York, NY 10016

INDEX